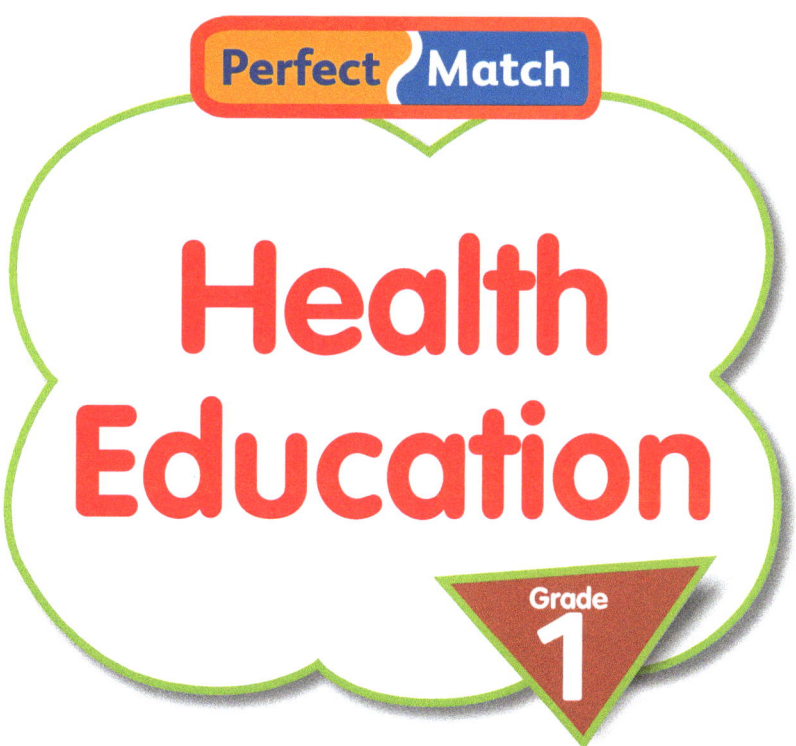

Dr Michael Chia

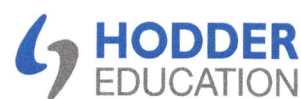

Hachette UK's policy is to use papers that are natural, renewable and recyclable products and made from wood grown in well-managed forests and other controlled sources. The logging and manufacturing processes are expected to conform to the environmental regulations of the country of origin.

ISBN: 978 981 47 6772 9

© Dr Michael Chia 2007, 2018

First published in 2007 by Pearson Education South Asia Pte Ltd

This new edition published in 2018 by
Hachette Singapore Private Limited
Published from 2023 by Hodder Education,
An Hachette UK Company
Carmelite House
50 Victoria Embankment
London EC4Y 0DZ
www.hoddereducation.com

Impression number   10 9 8 7 6 5
Year   2023

All rights reserved. Apart from any use permitted under UK copyright law, no part of this publication may be reproduced or transmitted in any form or by any means, electronic or mechanical, including photocopying and recording, or held within any information storage and retrieval system, without permission in writing from the publisher or under licence from the Copyright Licensing Agency Limited. Further details of such licences (for reprographic reproduction) may be obtained from the Copyright Licensing Agency Limited, www.cla.co.uk

Printed in Singapore

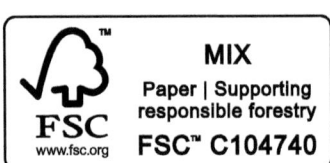

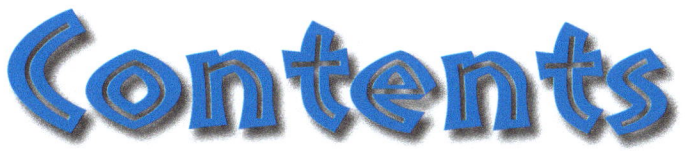

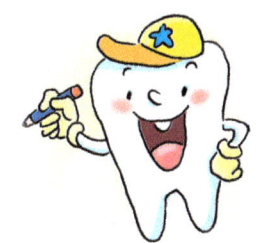

Physical Health

Lesson	Title	Page
1	Members Of The Body	3
2	Taller and Heavier	5
3	When I Grow Up …	9
4	Keeping Fit	13
5	Practise Good Posture	15
6 & 7	Nice And Clean	17
8	Treasure Your Teeth	21
9 & 10	Caring For My Mouth	23

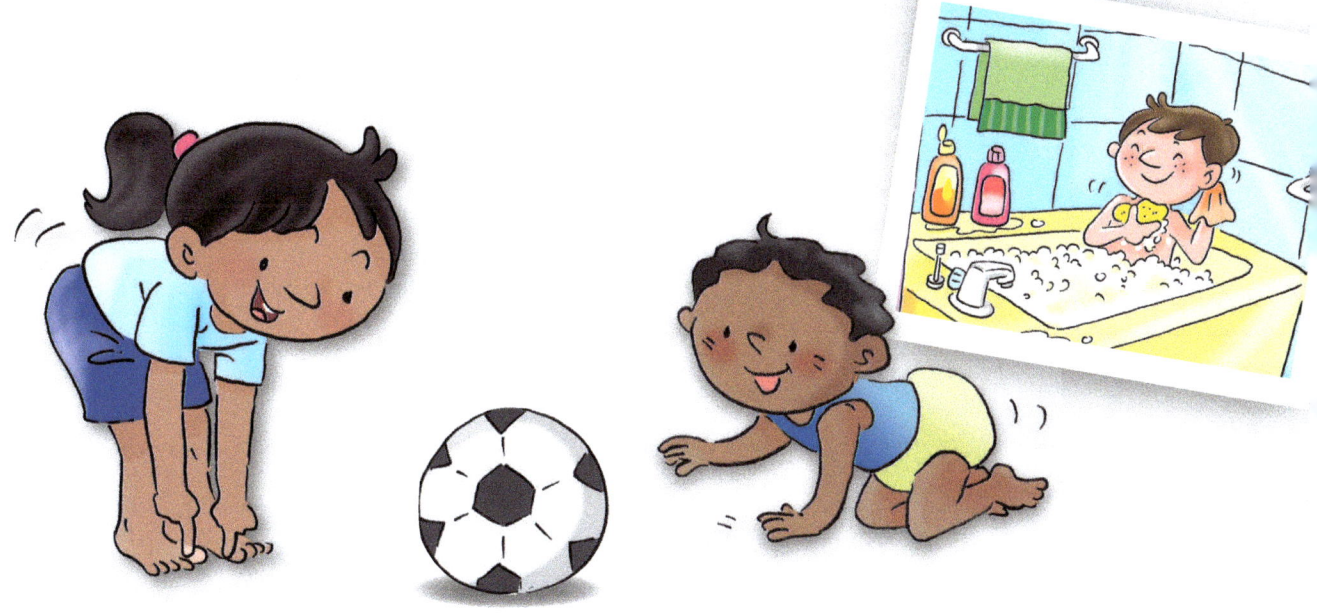

Environment And Your Health

Lesson	Title	Page
1	Watch Out!	29
2	Fire, Fire!	31
3	Not Water Play	33
4	Where Do I Cross?	35
5	Danger!	37
6	Going Home Alone	39
7	Be Aware!	41
8	Should I Go With Them?	43

Emotional And Psychological Health

Lesson	Title	Page
1	Feelings	47
2	How Do I Feel?	51
3	In A New Place	53
4	May I Touch You?	55
5	It Is Not My Fault	57
6	What Can I Do?	59
7	Being Safe At Home	61
8	Being Safe In Public	63

Learning Log   65-70

Introduction to the Pupil's Book

The **Perfect Match** Primary Health Education Pupil's Book is a full-colour textbook-cum-activity book. It contains lessons based on topics from the three dimensions in Health Education: Physical Health, Environment and Your Health, and Emotional and Psychological Health.

The book is organised by dimension and is presented in the order stated above. The pages in each dimension are colour-coded for easy reference.

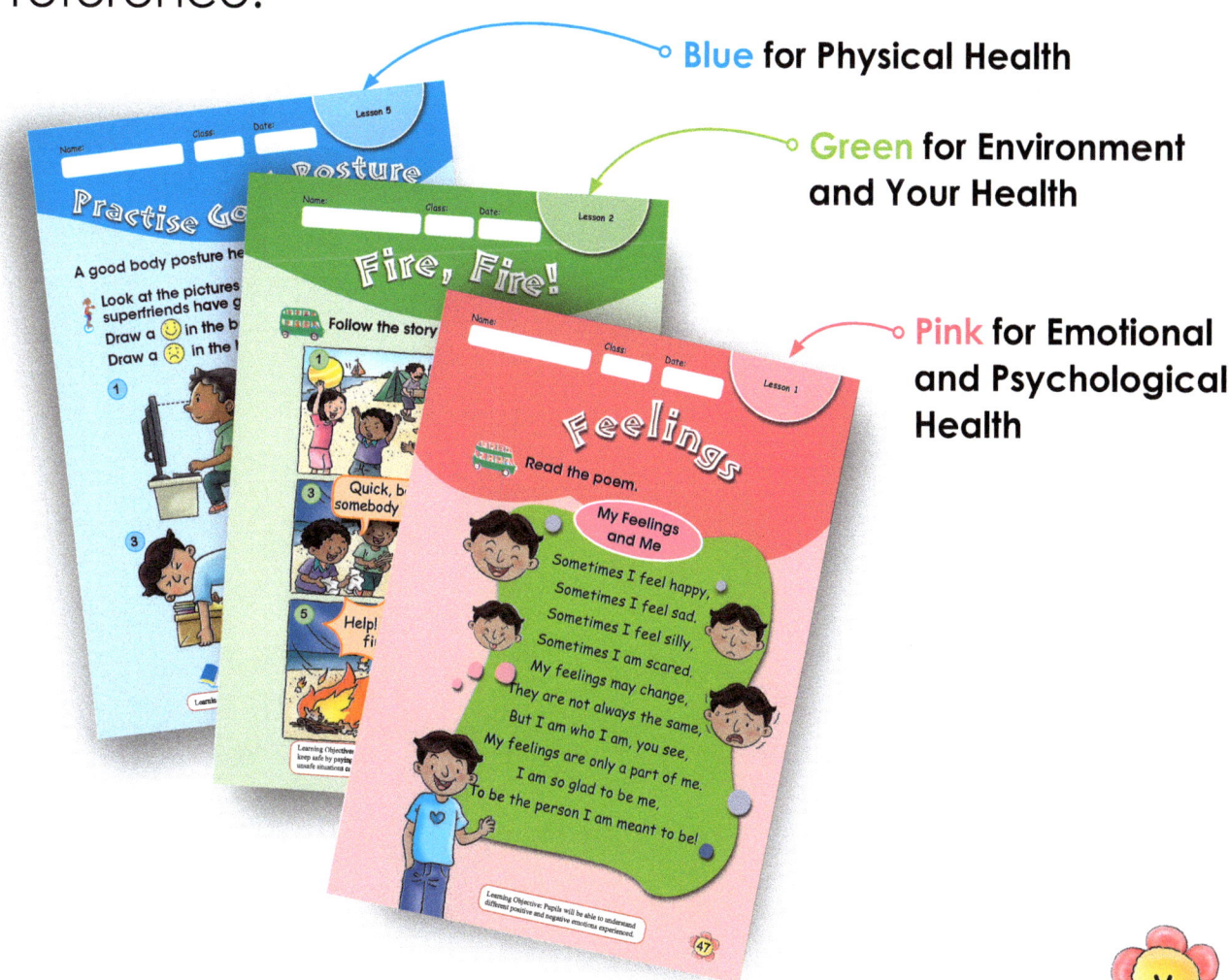

- **Blue** for Physical Health
- **Green** for Environment and Your Health
- **Pink** for Emotional and Psychological Health

The Pupil's Book contains a variety of activities such as role plays, surveys, songs, matching exercises and craft work. In addition, there is a mix of activities requiring work in pairs, in groups or with the class.

Four icons indicate the nature of the activity to be conducted.

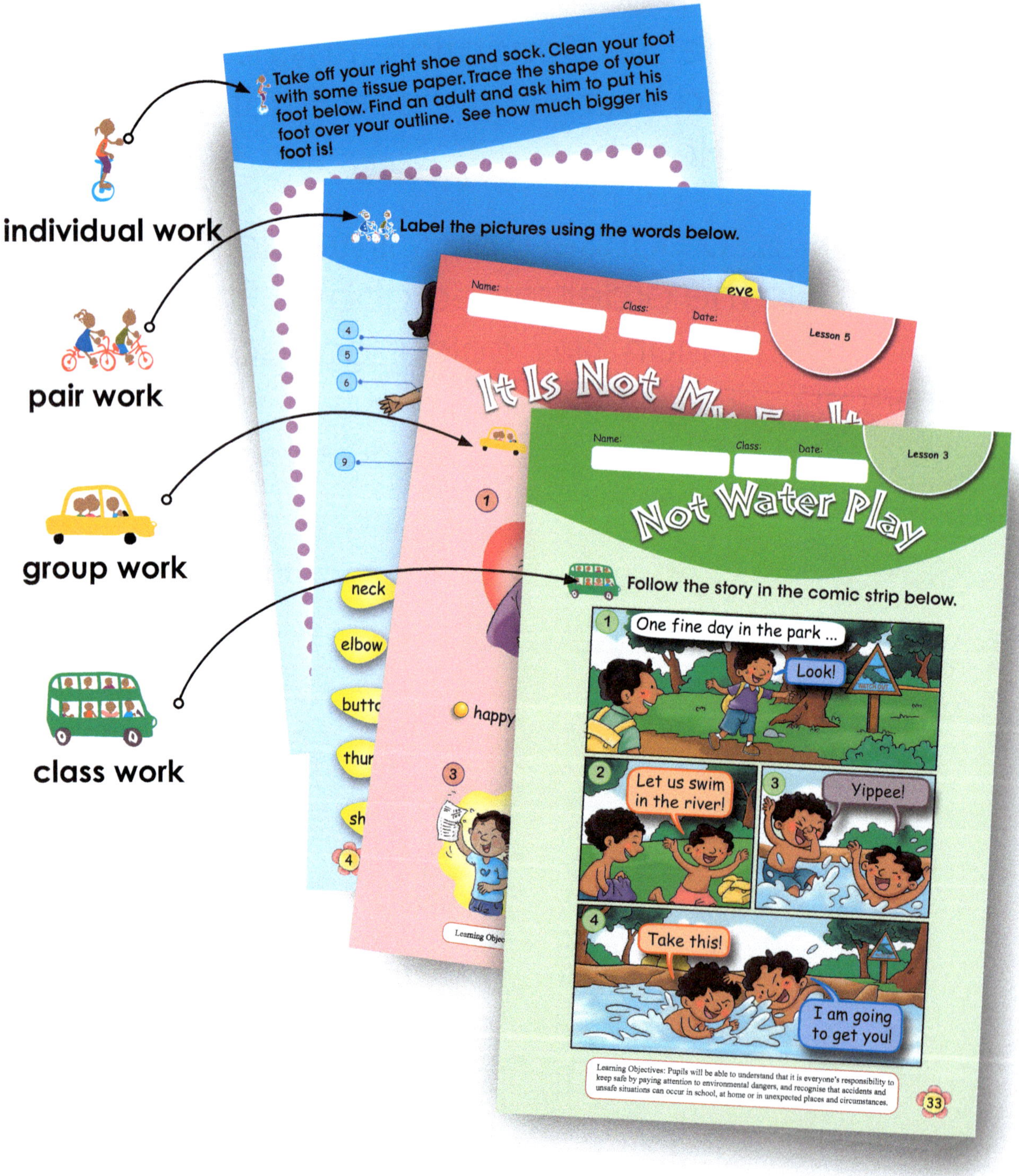

- individual work
- pair work
- group work
- class work

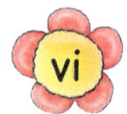

Difficult terms mentioned in the text are explained through a feature signalled by the dictionary icon.

The learning objective(s) for each lesson is/are listed for parents' and teachers' reference.

A dictionary icon signals the explanation of any difficult term(s) found on the page

The learning objective(s) for each lesson is/are indicated at the opening page of each lesson.

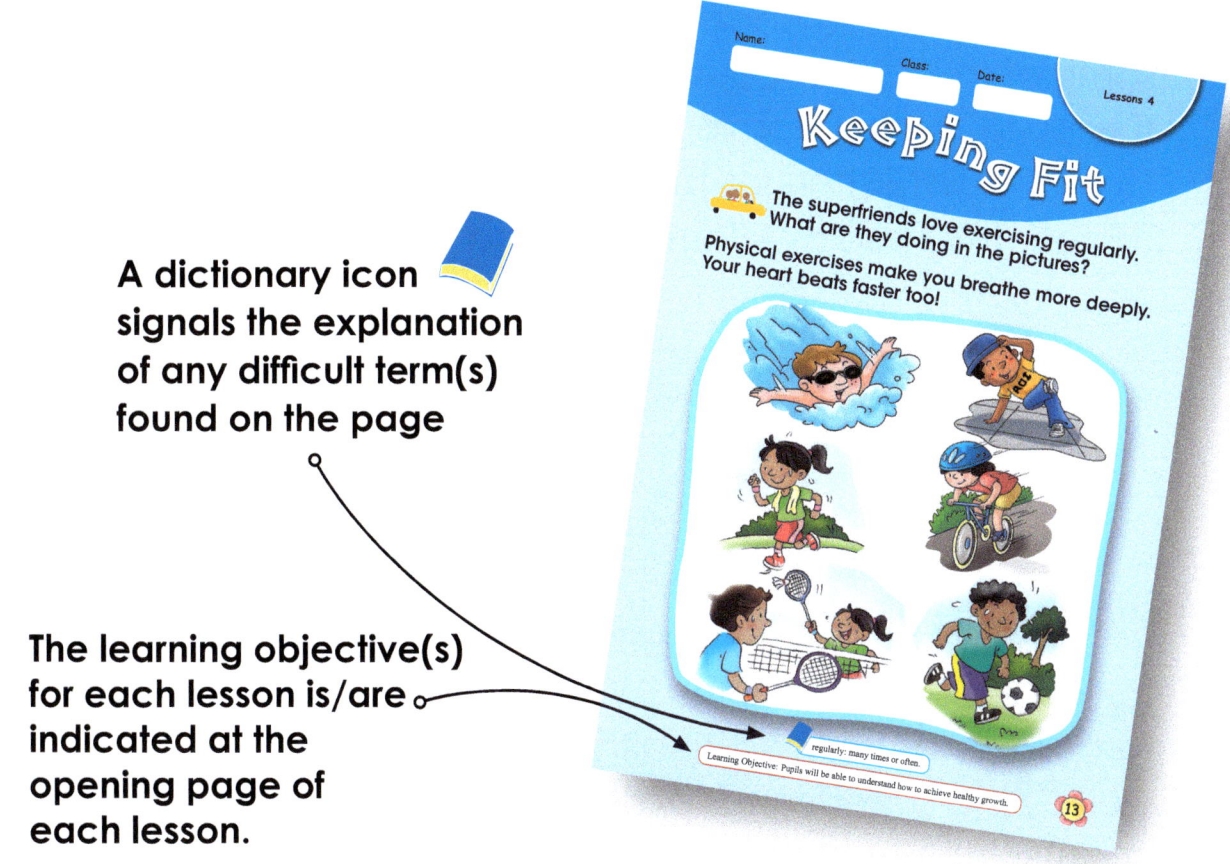

A Note on Short Forms: In the first three books, short-forms of verbs are avoided as early users of the language may not have knowledge of them. In Books 4, 5 and 6, these contractions are present throughout so that the language flows more naturally and pupils can become more acquainted with real English use.

A Learning Log has been added at the end of the book to give opportunity for reflective learning.

Meet the Superfriends

The materials in the Perfect Match **Perfect Match** Primary Health Education Pupil's Book revolve around six superfriends from some of the ASEAN countries. These six friends will accompany the pupils in the learning process as they move from Book 1 to 6. The first letters of their names — Haris, Eileen, Ajit, Lam, Tawan and Harold — form the word 'h-e-a-l-t-h'.

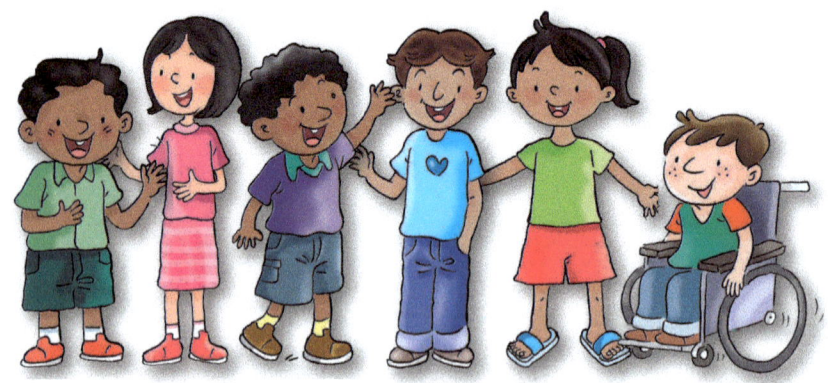

Taking the cue from the World Health Organization (WHO) to build 'a better and healthier future for people all over the world', the superfriends come together from different ASEAN countries to help young people like themselves develop healthy habits to ensure a better future. This health series aims to help pupils start early in health education, to keep themselves well physically, psychologically and emotionally. In addition, they will also learn to behave responsibly in order to enhance the environment in their home countries.

Hi, I am Haris.

Haris is a well-built Malaysian boy. He is the wise one among the superfriends. He is fun and peace-loving and tries his best to keep the people around him happy.

"Hi, I am Eileen."

Eileen is a tall slim Singaporean girl. She loves Maths and Science and knows a lot about computers. Eileen enjoys helping her friends with school work.

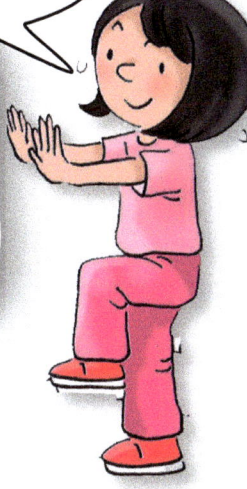

"Hi, I am Ajit."

Ajit is a Malaysian boy who loves reading and has a flair for languages. He speaks well and is always eager to listen to his friends when they have problems.

"Hi, I am Lam."

Lam is a Vietnamese boy who is active and full of ideas. He loves school and hopes to be a teacher when he grows up. He is good-natured and patient and is extremely well-liked.

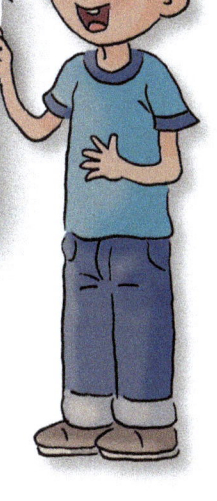

"Hi, I am Tawan."

Tawan is an athletic and sporty Thai girl who also loves art. She is the most physically active and well-rounded person in the group. She is smart and strong in character but also fun-loving and witty.

"Hi, I am Harold."

Harold has a Canadian father and a biracial mother who is half Singaporean. He is musically talented and has great willpower. Despite his disability, he has never felt disadvantaged and he always encourages his friends to pursue their interests.

About The Author

Dr Michael Chia is Professor of Paediatric Exercise Science at the Physical Education & Sports Science Group in the National Institute of Education (NIE), Nanyang Technological University (NTU). He is an established author in the field of Health Education, Physical Education and Sports Science.

His health education publications include *Healthy, Well and Wise: Take PRIDE For A Life of Wellness*, *Invest in Better Health* and *Treks: All Aboard!*.

Physical Health

In this section, you will learn:

- about your body and how it changes as you grow;

- how exercise, water, fresh air and sunshine are good for you;

- how to keep your body clean; and

- how to take good care of your teeth, gums and tongue.

Name: Class: Date: Lesson 1

Members Of The Body

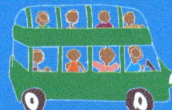 Sing the song below.

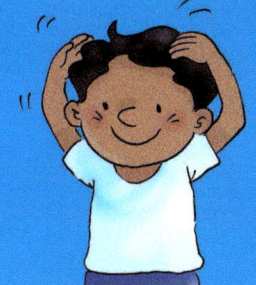

My Body

Verse 1:
Head and shoulders,
knees and toes,
Knees and toes, knees
and toes!
Heads and shoulders,
knees and toes,
Members of my body!

Verse 3:
Neck and chest, and
hips and legs
Hips and legs, hips and
legs!
Neck and chest, and
hips and legs
Members of my body!

Verse 2:
Elbows, ankles,
feet and soles
Feet and soles,
feet and soles!
Elbows, ankles,
feet and soles
Members of my body!

Verse 4
Eyes and ears, and
mouth and nose,
Mouth and nose, mouth
and nose!
Eyes and ears, and
mouth and nose,
Members of my body!

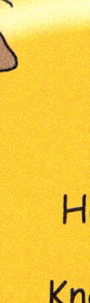
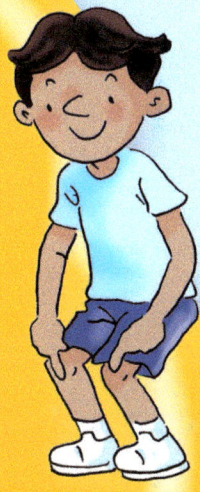
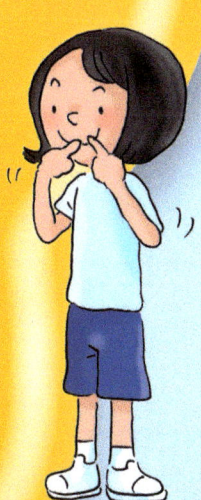
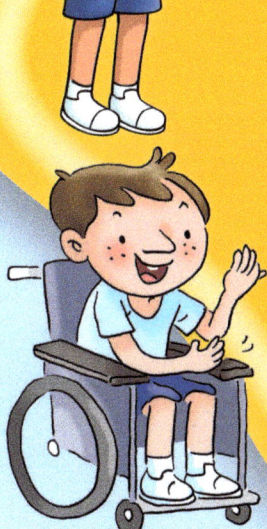

Learning Objective: Pupils will be able to recognise the different stages of growth and development of their bodies.

3

Label the pictures using the words below.

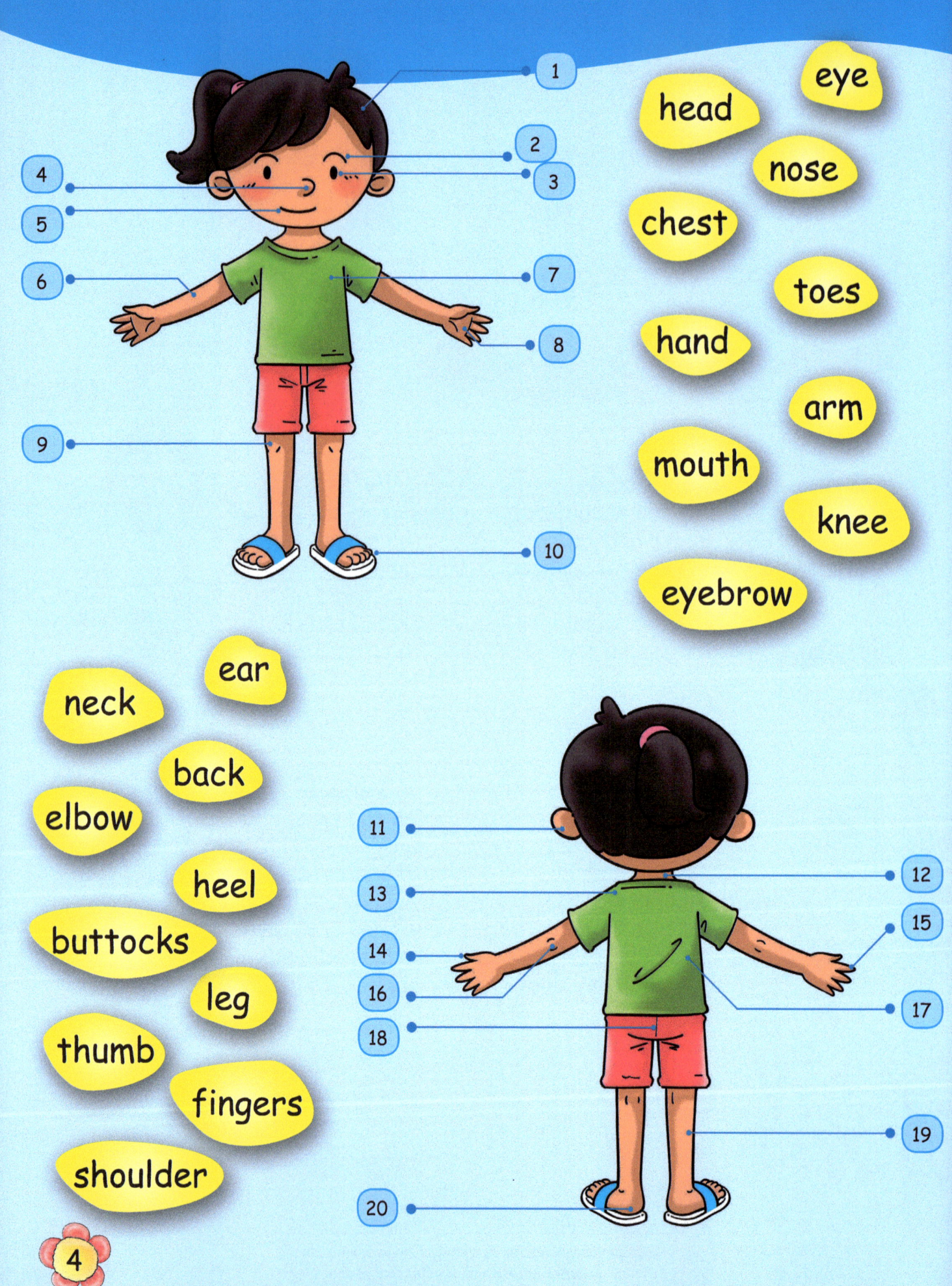

Taller And Heavier

Name: Class: Date: Lesson 2

Look at the superfriends when they were super babies!

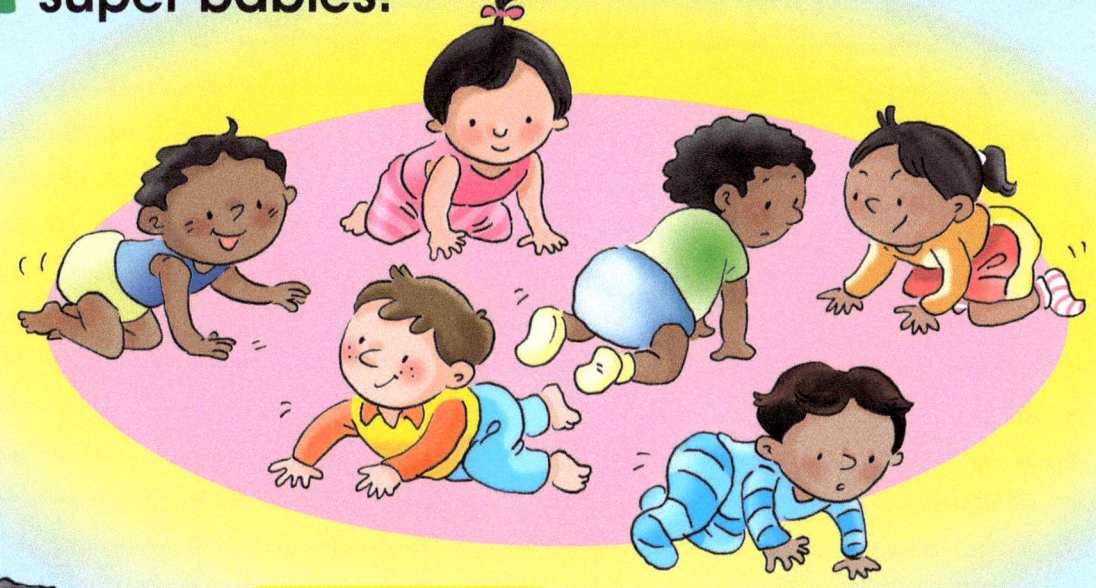

We were much smaller then!

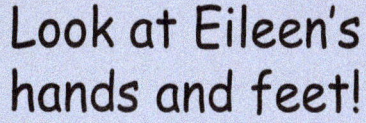

We were so cute!

Look at Eileen's hands and feet!

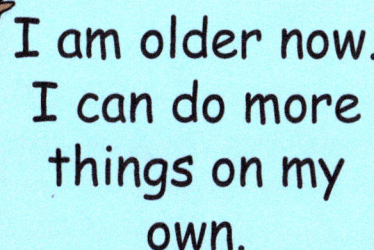

I am older now. I can do more things on my own.

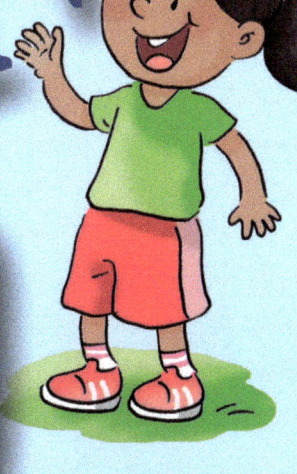

Learning Objective: Pupils will be able to recognise the different stages of growth and development of their bodies.

As you grow, you will change in many ways. You will grow taller and heavier. You will also learn new things.

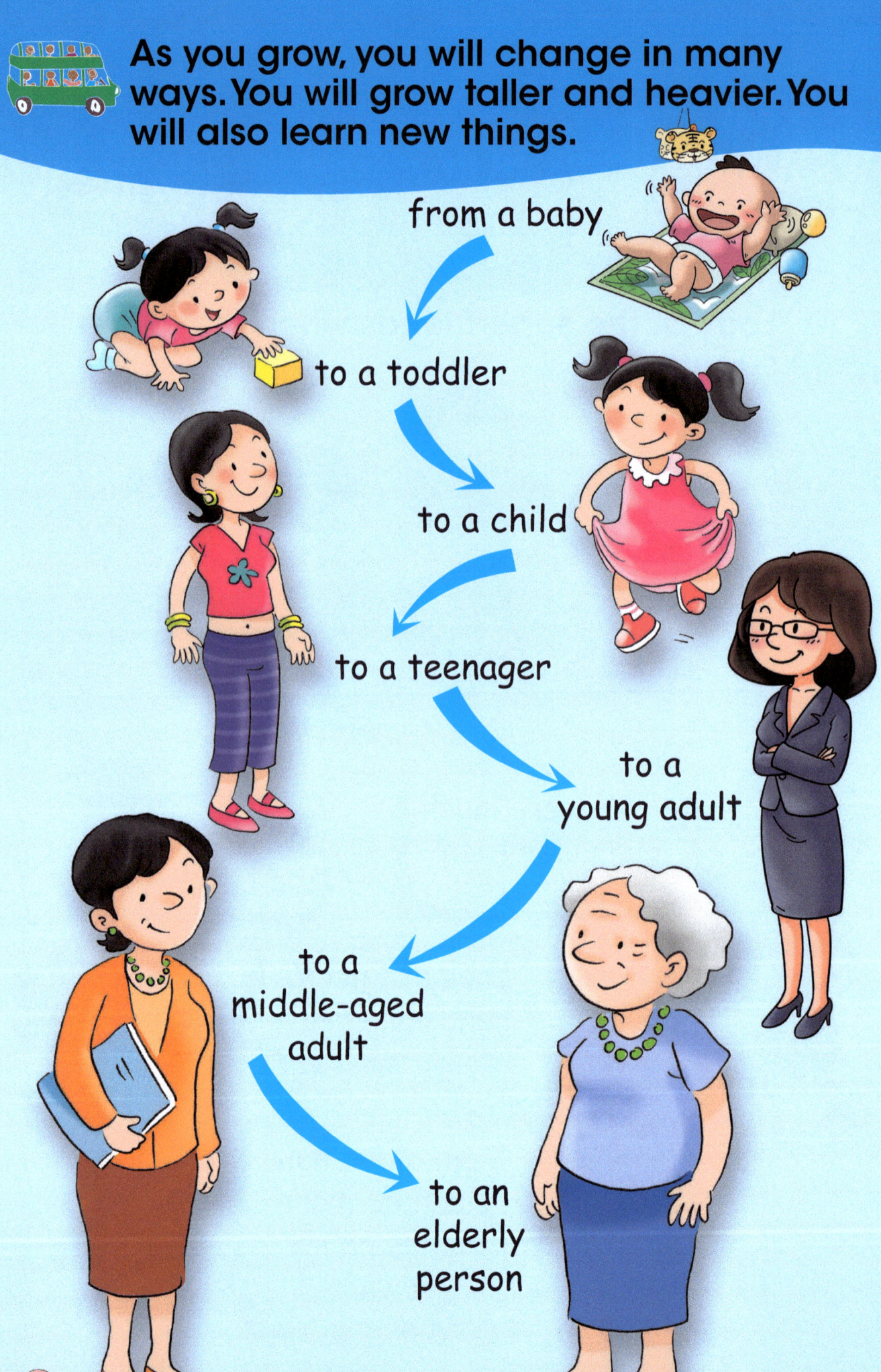

from a baby
to a toddler
to a child
to a teenager
to a young adult
to a middle-aged adult
to an elderly person

What are some things you can do now which you could not do as a baby? Write them down in the spaces below.

Two things I could not do as a baby ...

Three things I can do on my own now ...

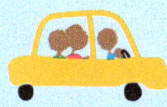 **Talk about what you have written in the two boxes with your friends.**

Take off your right shoe and sock. Clean your foot with some tissue paper. Trace the shape of your foot below. Find an adult and ask him to put his foot over your outline. See how much bigger his foot is!

Name: Class: Date: Lesson 3

When I Grow Up...

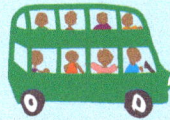 **Read what the superfriends are saying. What do they want to be when they grow up?**

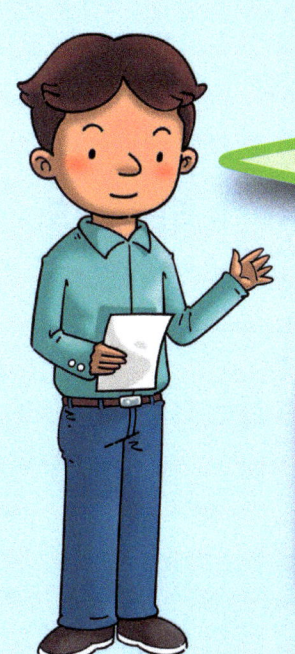

"I want to be a teacher so that I can help young people learn."

"I want to be a nurse. I hope to help people who are ill get better."

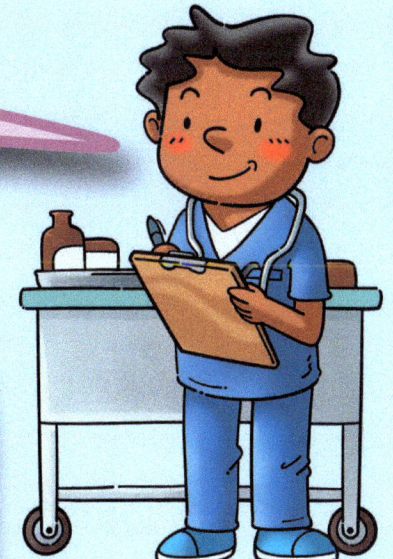

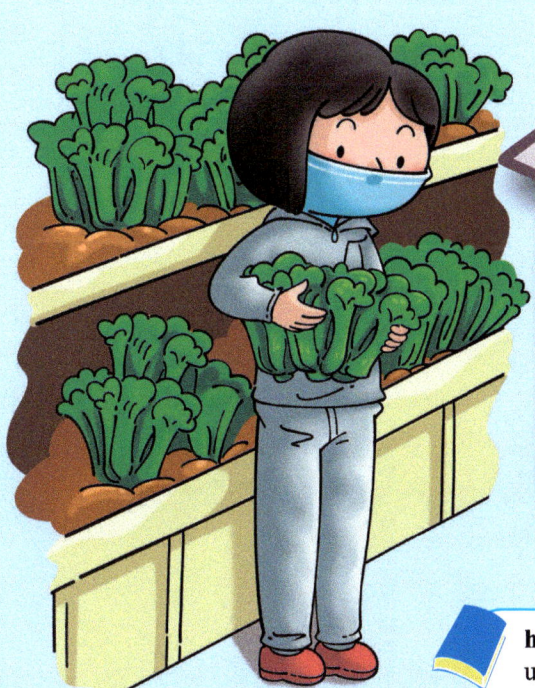

"I want to be a high-tech farmer and grow more food. My farms will be friendly to the environment."

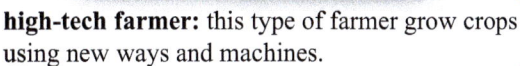 **high-tech farmer:** this type of farmer grow crops using new ways and machines.

Learning Objective: Pupils will be able to recognise the different stages of growth and development of their bodies.

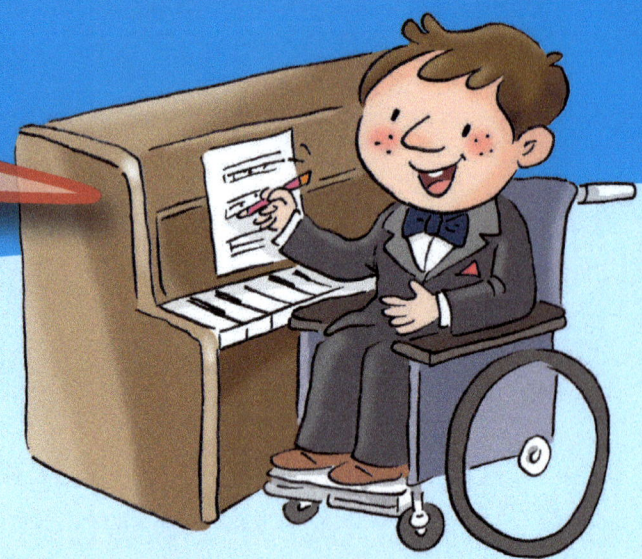

"I like music. Should I be a singer, a songwriter or a performer?"

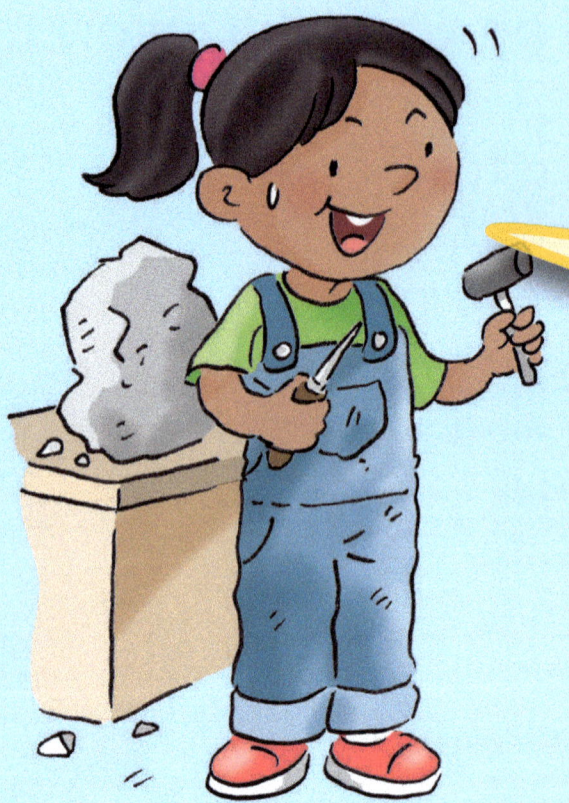

"I enjoy art and I want to create beautiful art pieces. Perhaps I can be a sculptor!"

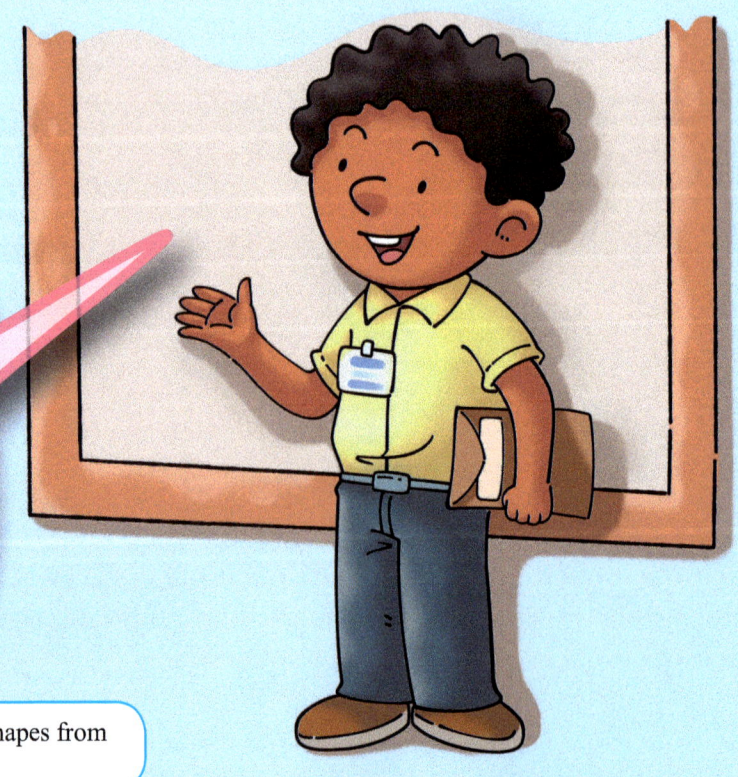

"I want to be a social worker. People with problems can come to me for help."

sculptor: an artist who makes new shapes from stone, wood or metal.

What do your classmates want to be when they grow up?

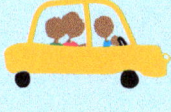 **Ask two classmates what they want to be when they grow up. Write their answers in the spaces below.**

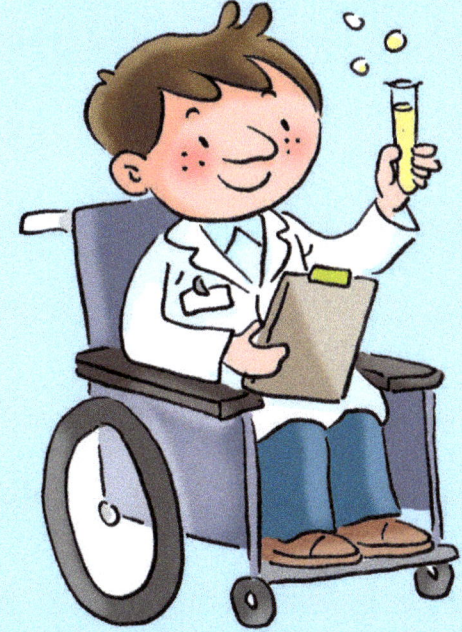

My friend's name is

_____.

He/She wants to be

_____.

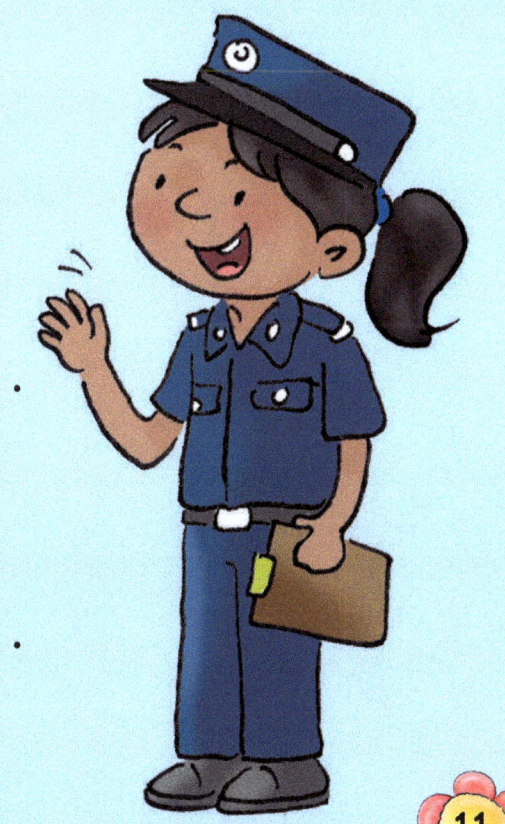

My friend's name is

_____.

He/She wants to be

_____.

What do you want to be when you grow up? Write and draw your answer in the space below.

I want to be _____ .

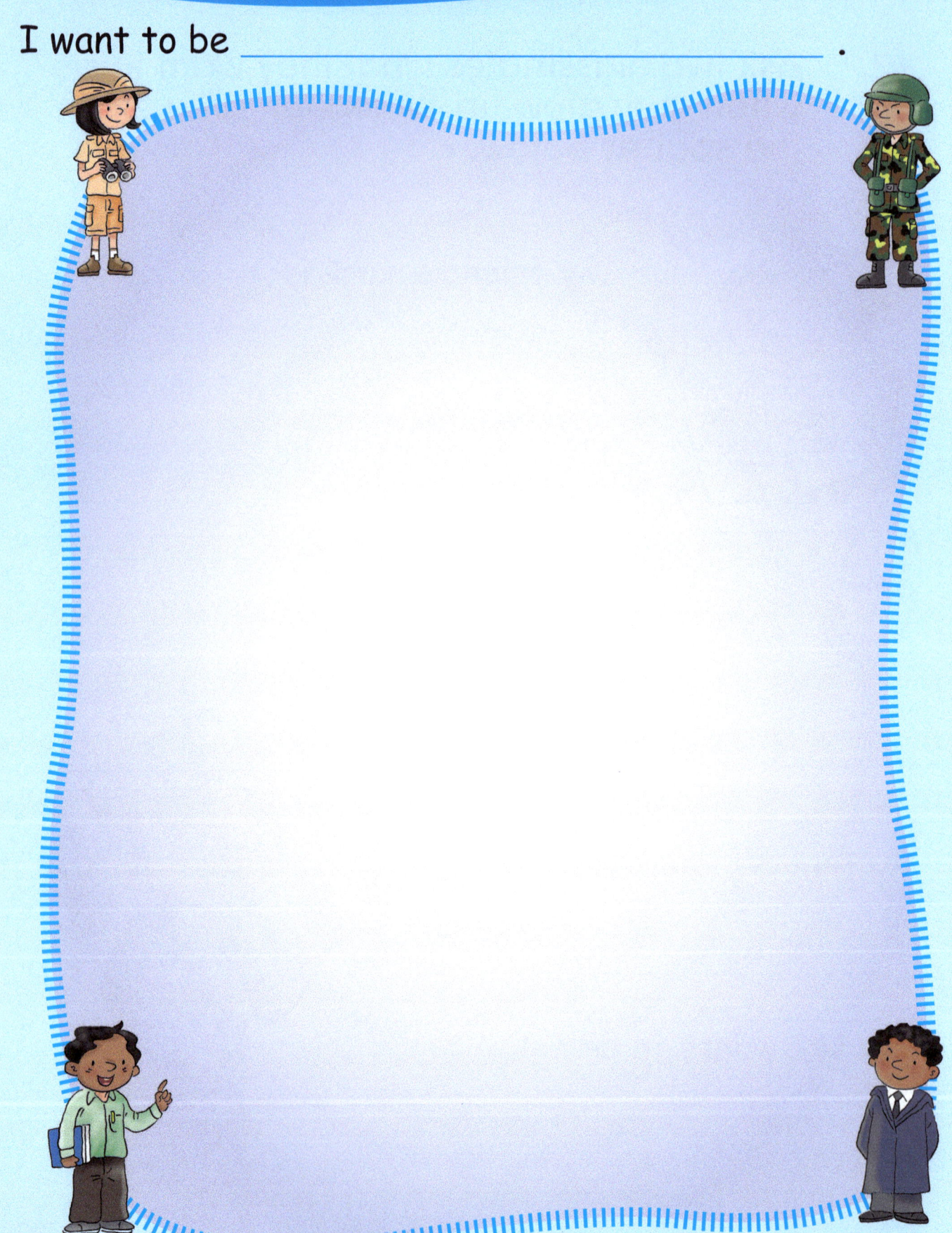

Name: Class: Date:

Lessons 4

Keeping Fit

🚗 The superfriends love exercising regularly. What are they doing in the pictures?

Physical exercises make you breathe more deeply. Your heart beats faster too!

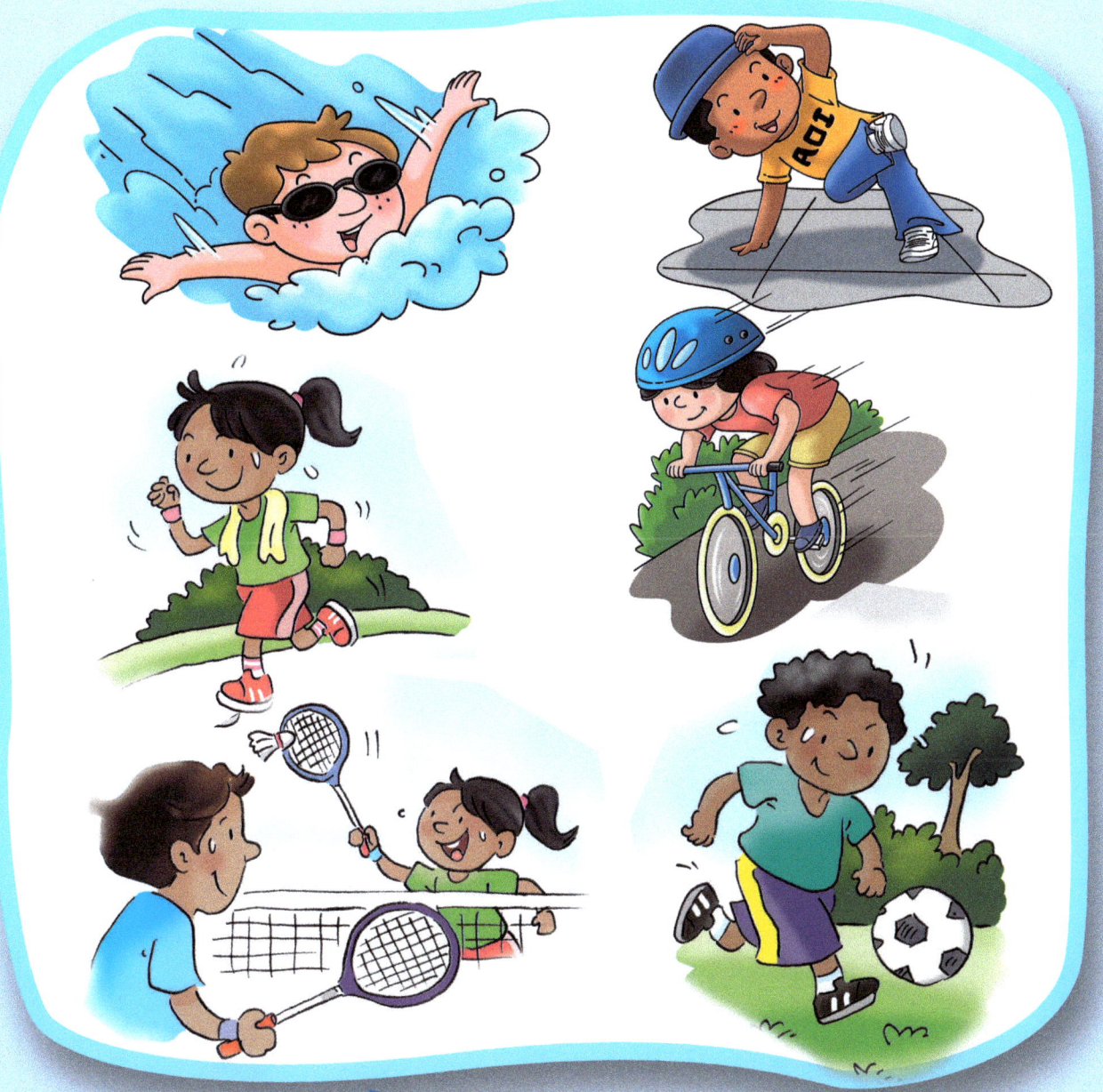

📘 **regularly:** many times or often.

Learning Objective: Pupils will be able to understand how to achieve healthy growth.

Exercising regularly is good for you. It keeps you healthy and helps you to grow well. After you exercise, remember to drink lots of water.

Circle the words that describe physical exercises.

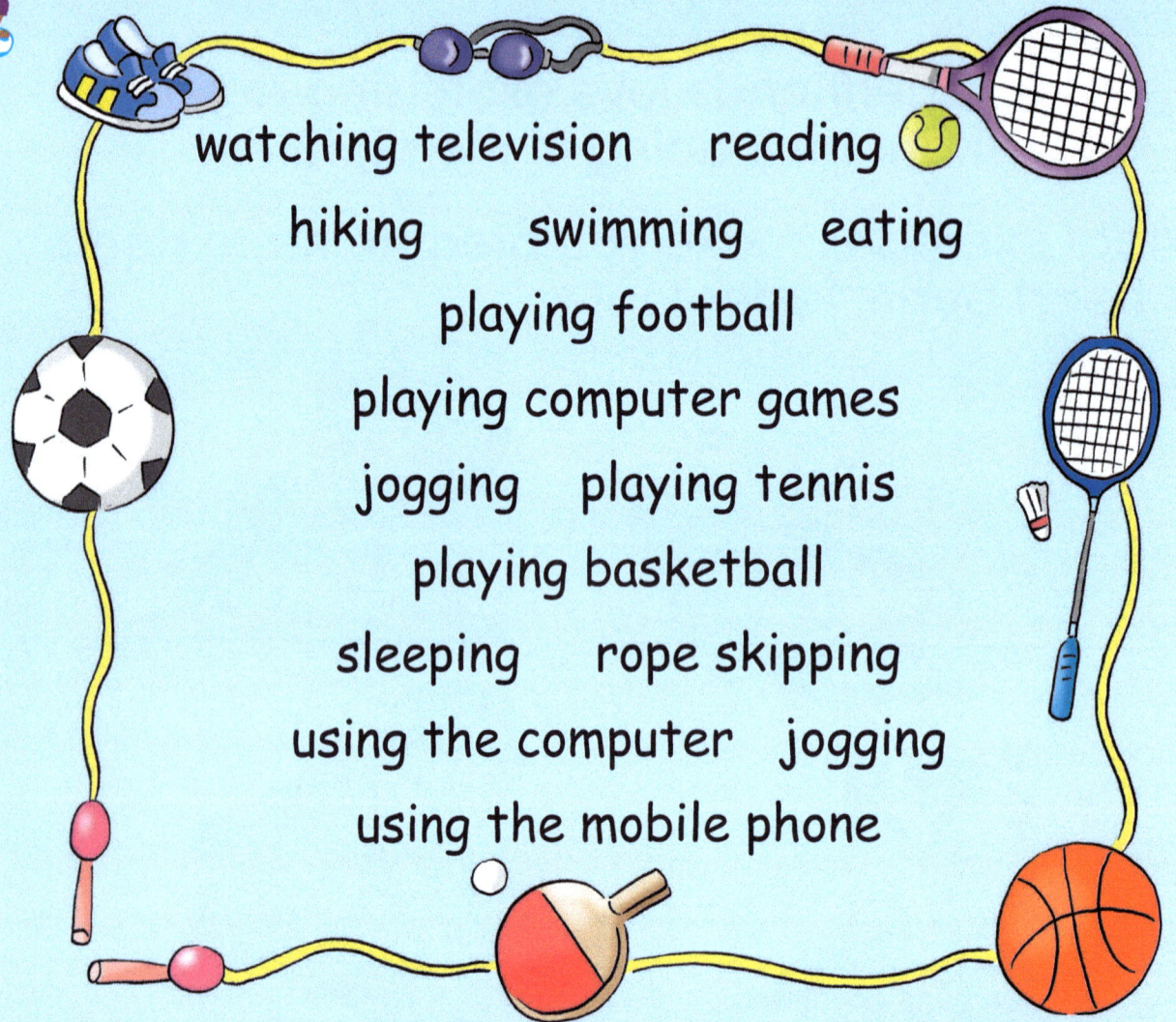

watching television   reading
hiking   swimming   eating
playing football
playing computer games
jogging   playing tennis
playing basketball
sleeping   rope skipping
using the computer   jogging
using the mobile phone

What are the activities you do *indoors* and *outdoors*? Start the list with the activities you enjoy most.

Indoor Activities	Outdoor Activities

Name: Class: Date: Lesson 5

Practise Good Posture

A good body posture helps us to grow well.

Look at the pictures below. Do the superfriends have good body postures?

Draw a 🙂 in the box if the posture is good.

Draw a ☹ in the box if the posture is poor.

1.

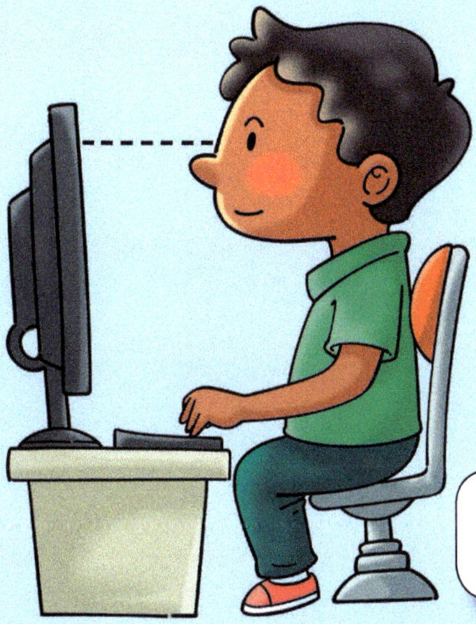

2.

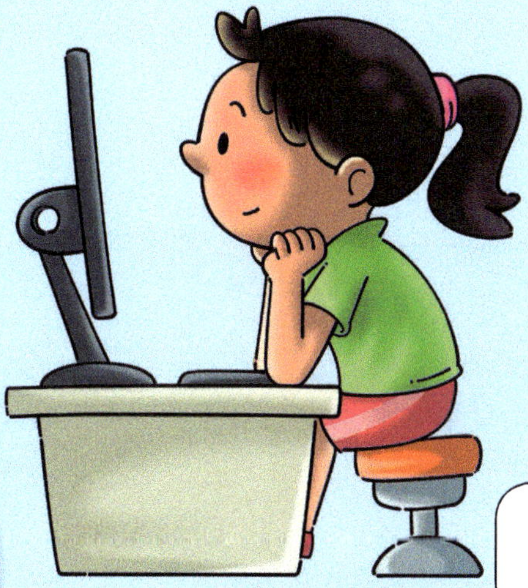

3.

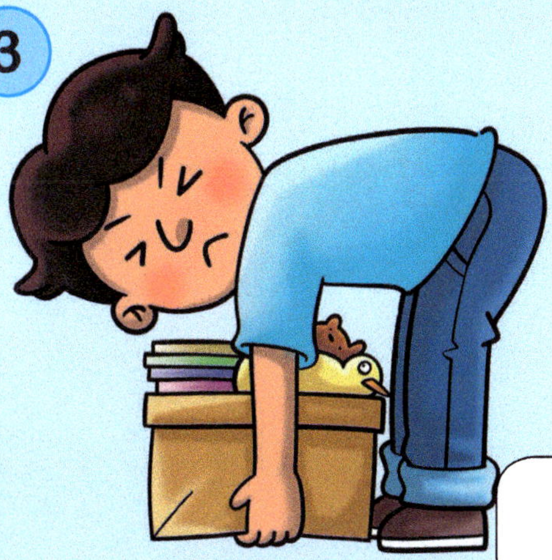

4.

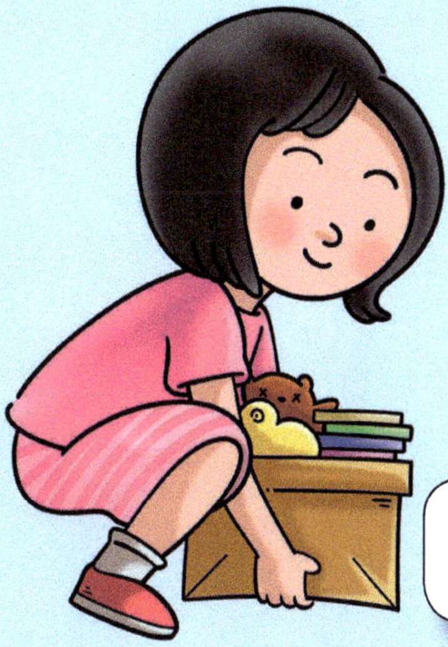

posture: the position you hold your body in when you sit or stand.

Learning Objective: Pupils will be able to understand how to achieve healthy growth.

15

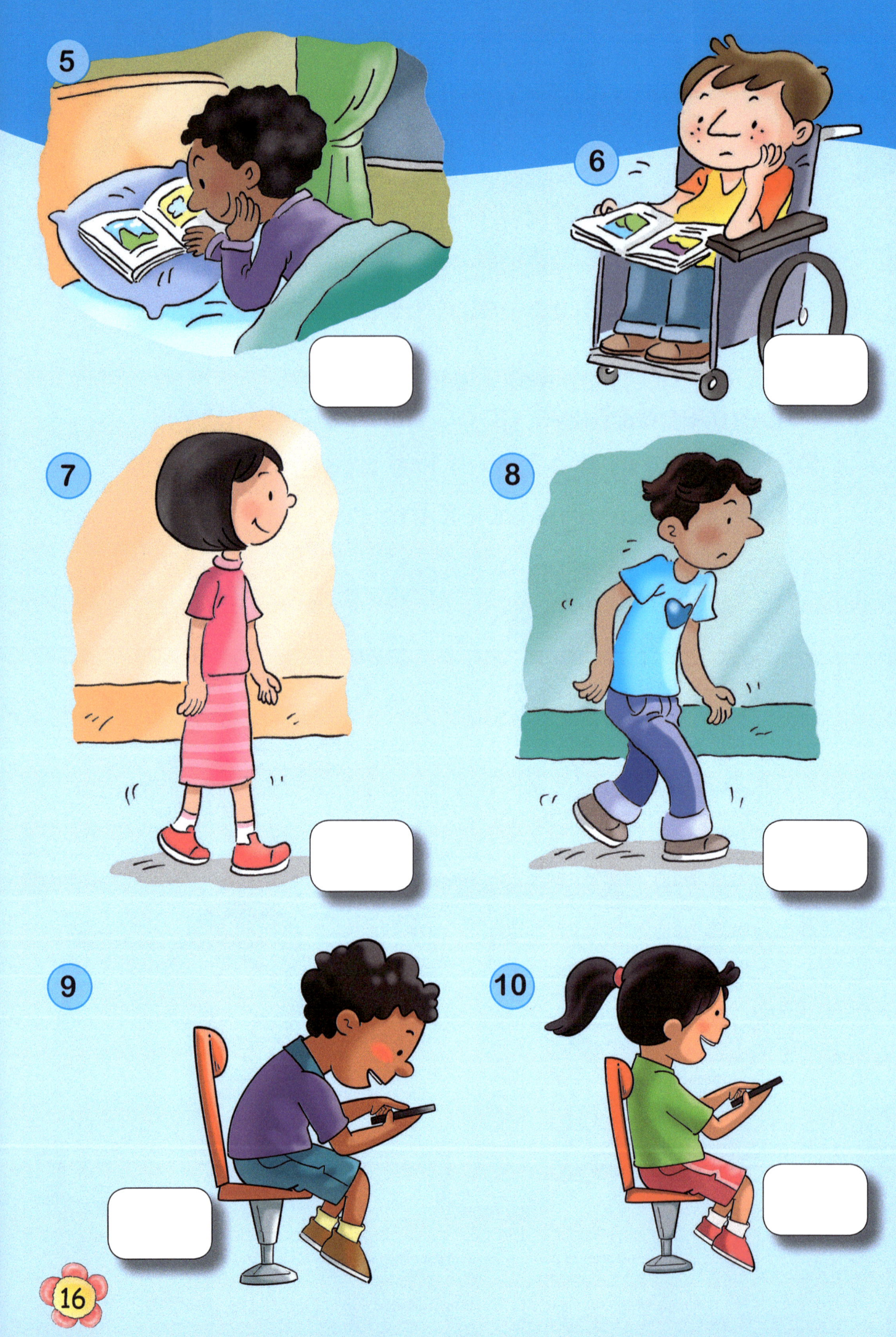

Name: Class: Date:

Lessons 6 & 7

Nice And Clean

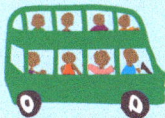 Look at the picture below. Read what Tawan, Eileen, Harold and Lam are saying.

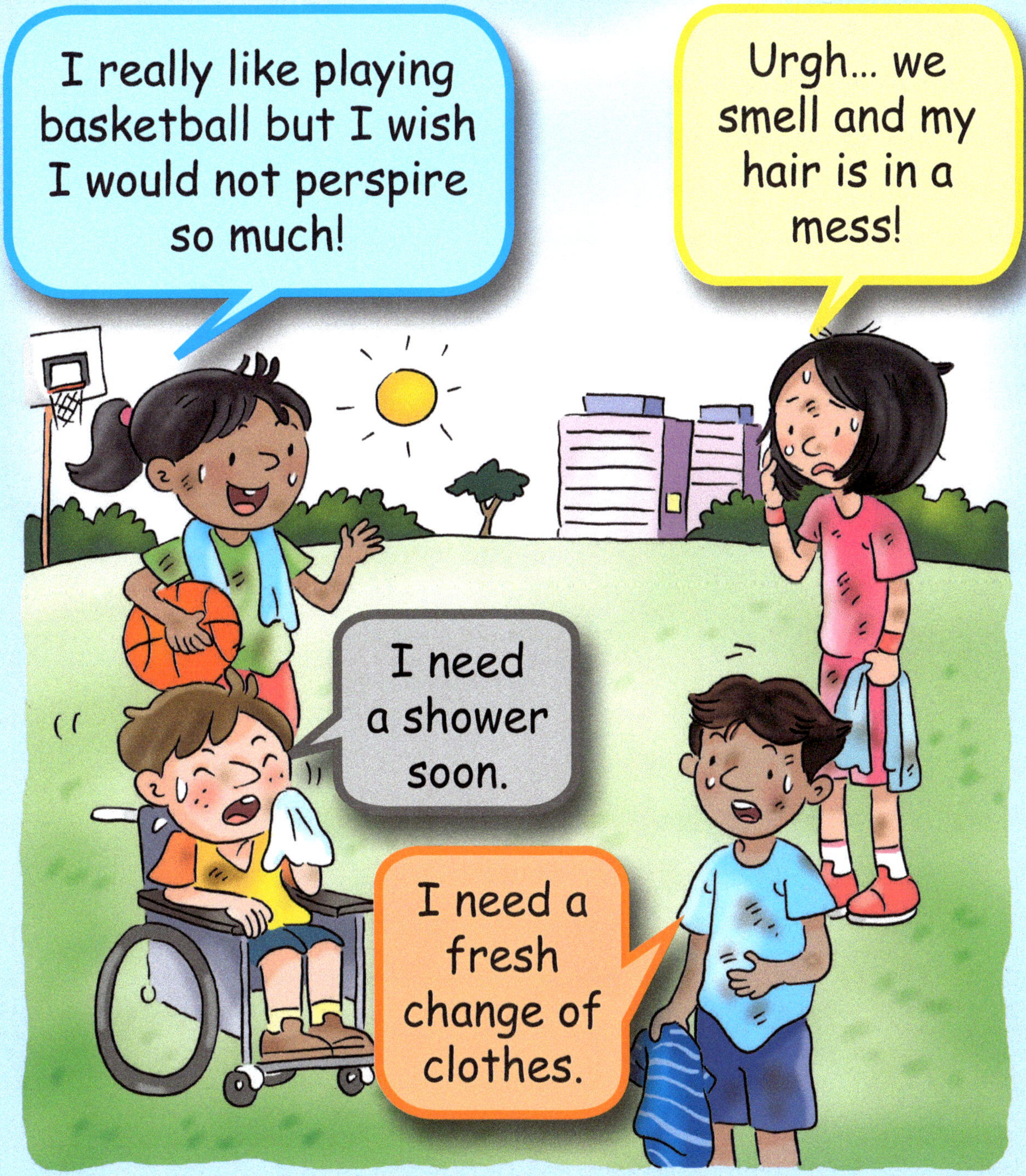

> I really like playing basketball but I wish I would not perspire so much!

> Urgh... we smell and my hair is in a mess!

> I need a shower soon.

> I need a fresh change of clothes.

Learning Objective: Pupils will be able to establish daily habits for caring for their bodies in order to maintain or improve health and prevent illnesses.

Practising good hygiene keeps your body clean. It also helps you stay healthy.

How do you practise good hygiene? Here are some ways.

Shower at least twice a day. Wash up after a physical activity too. Wash your face, neck, elbows, knees and toes. Clean behind your ears too.

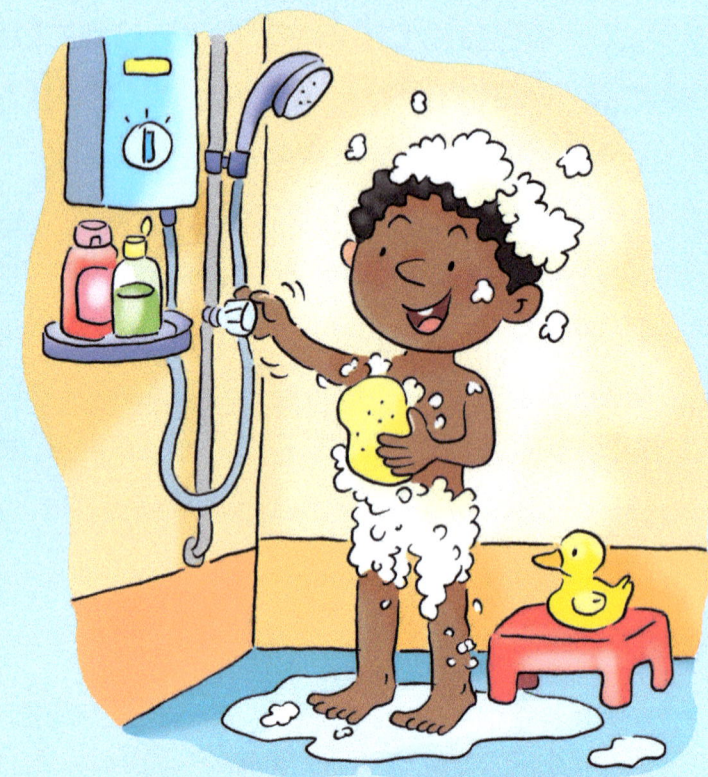

Do not waste water!

Is there a problem with using water in your town, city or village?

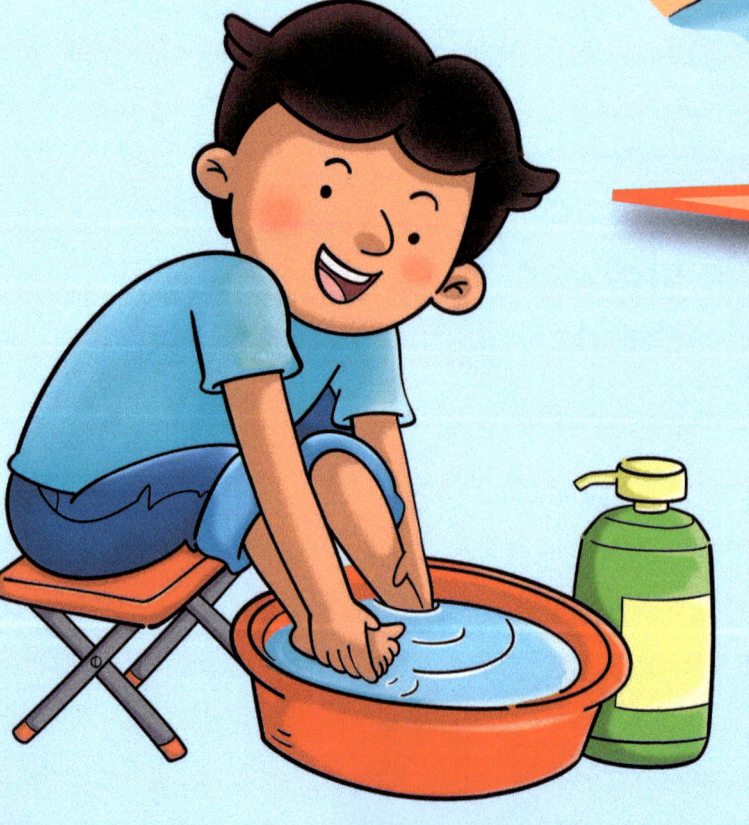

hygiene: the practice of keeping clean.

Wash your hands before and after meals, and when they are dirty.

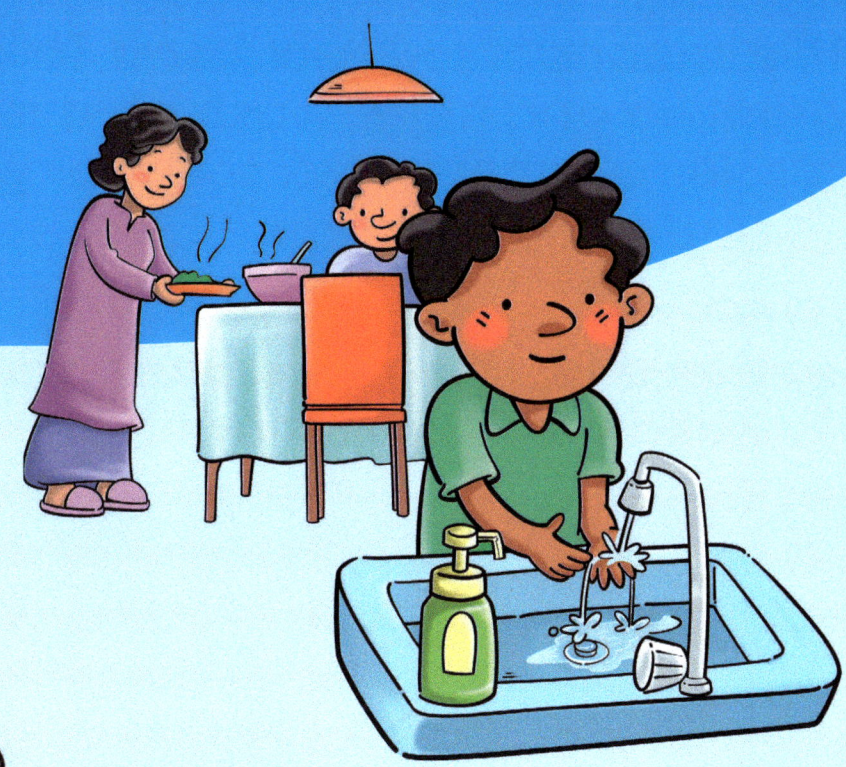

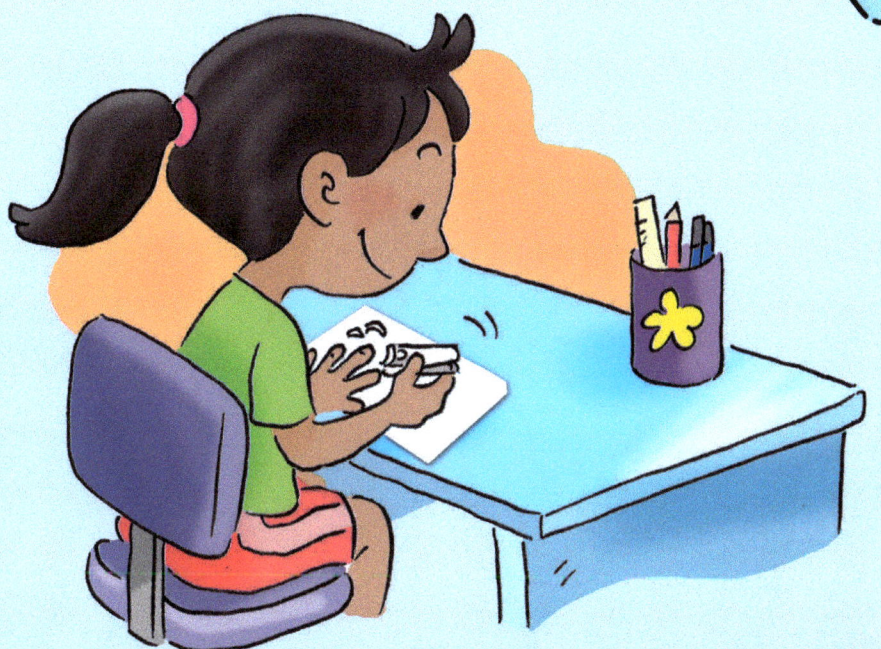

Keep your fingernails and toenails short.

Change your bedsheets and pillowcases regularly. Get enough sleep and wake up feeling fresh and rested.

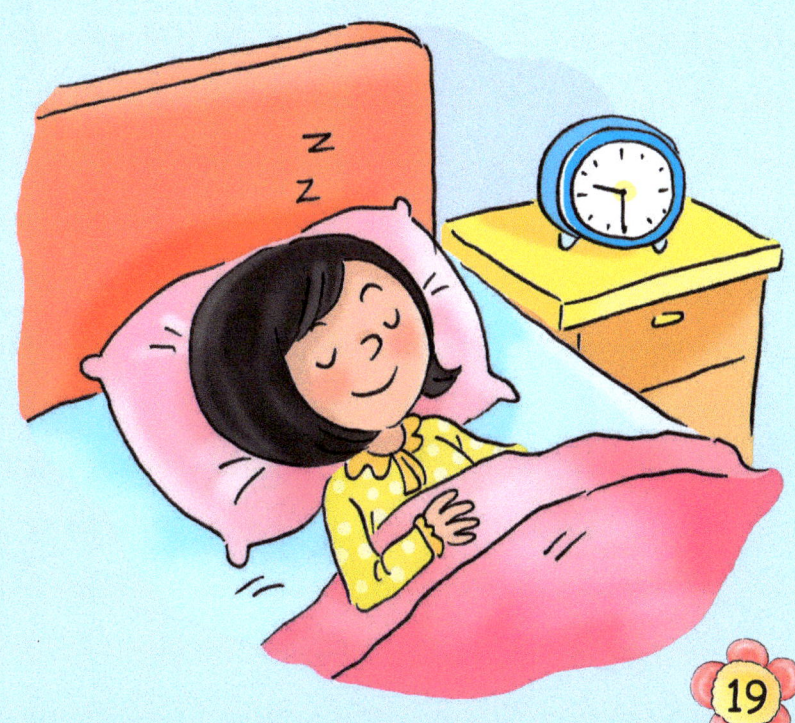

It is important to keep clean. Take a shower every morning and night. Wash up after exercising too. Remember to use soap for your body and shampoo for your hair.

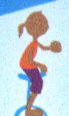 Circle the areas you must pay attention to when you take a shower.

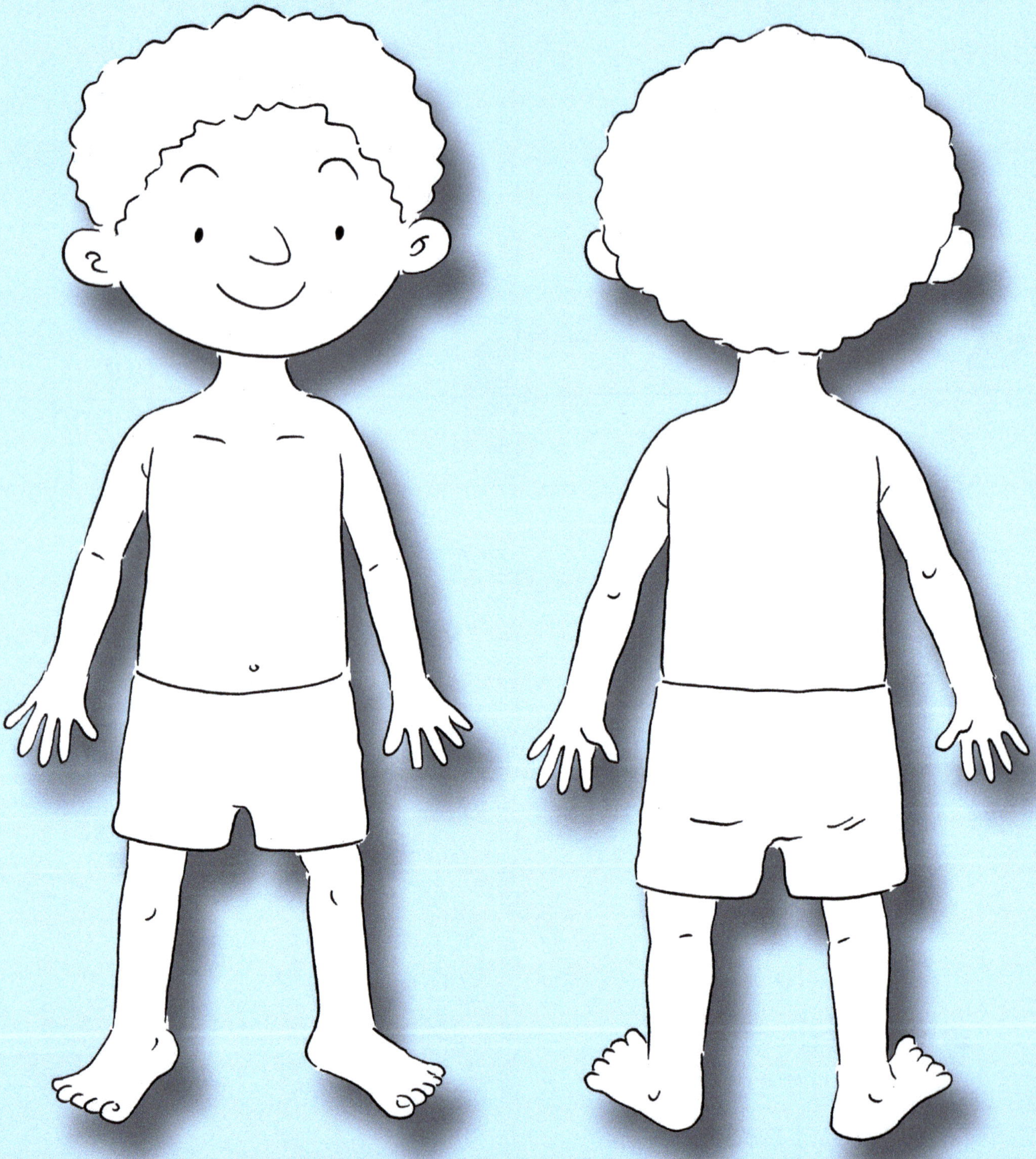

Name: Class: Date:

Lesson 8

Treasure Your Teeth

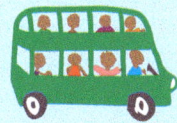 Follow the story in the comic strip below.

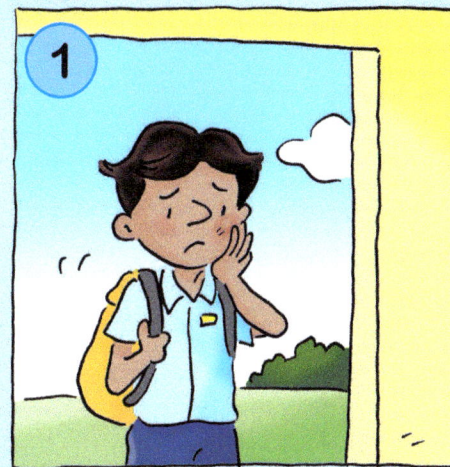
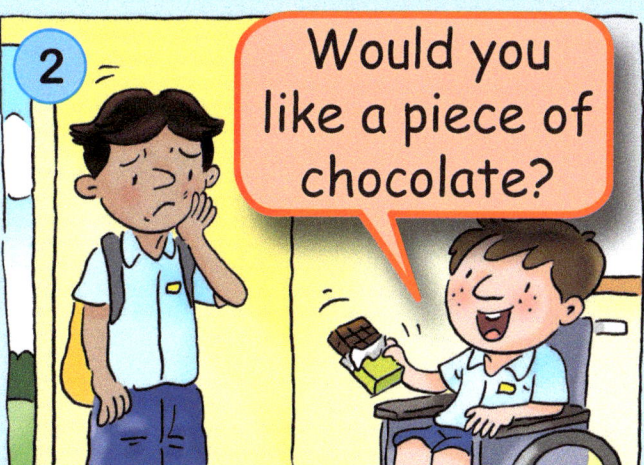
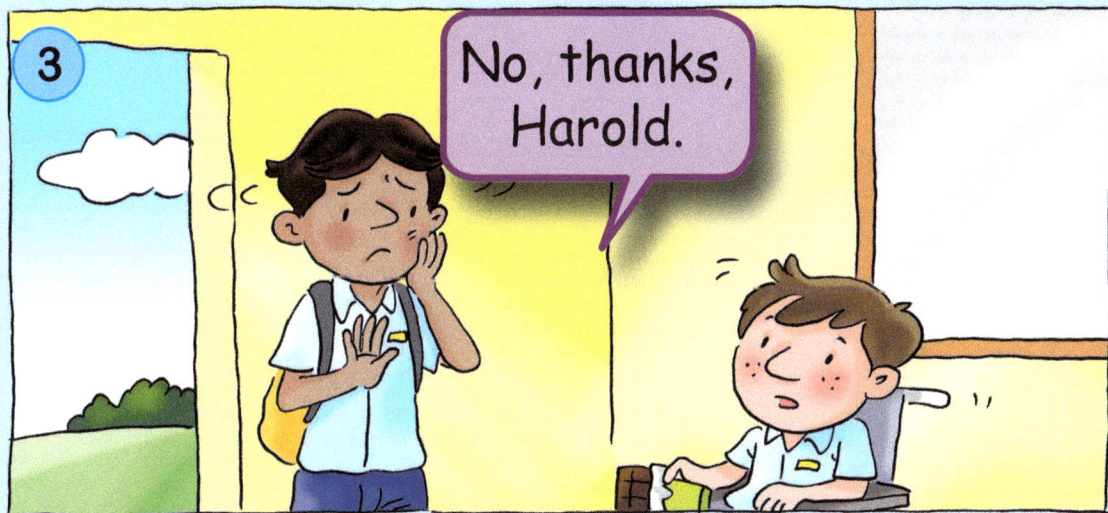
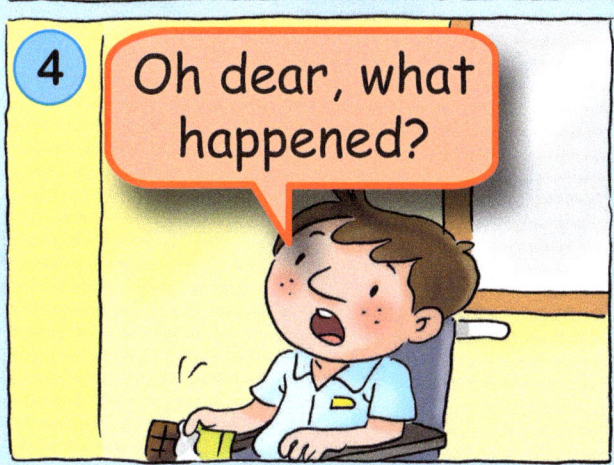
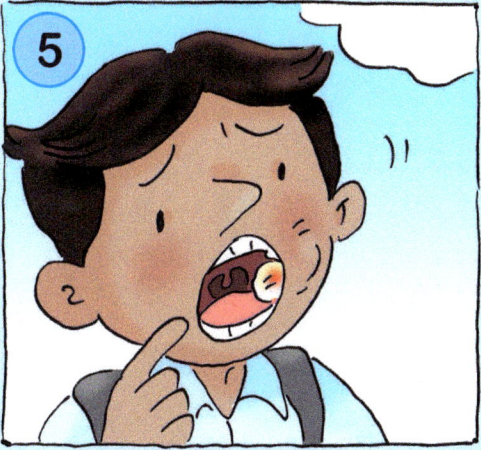

Learning Objective: Pupils will be able to recognise the importance of developing good oral hygiene habits to ensure that the teeth are healthy and well maintained.

Everyone has two sets of teeth. The first set is called milk teeth. Most of your teeth belong to the first set. When you lose your milk teeth, new ones will grow. These are your permanent teeth.

Have you lost any teeth before? Draw a cross (❌) on them in the picture below.

permanent: lasting, or supposed to last a long time or forever.

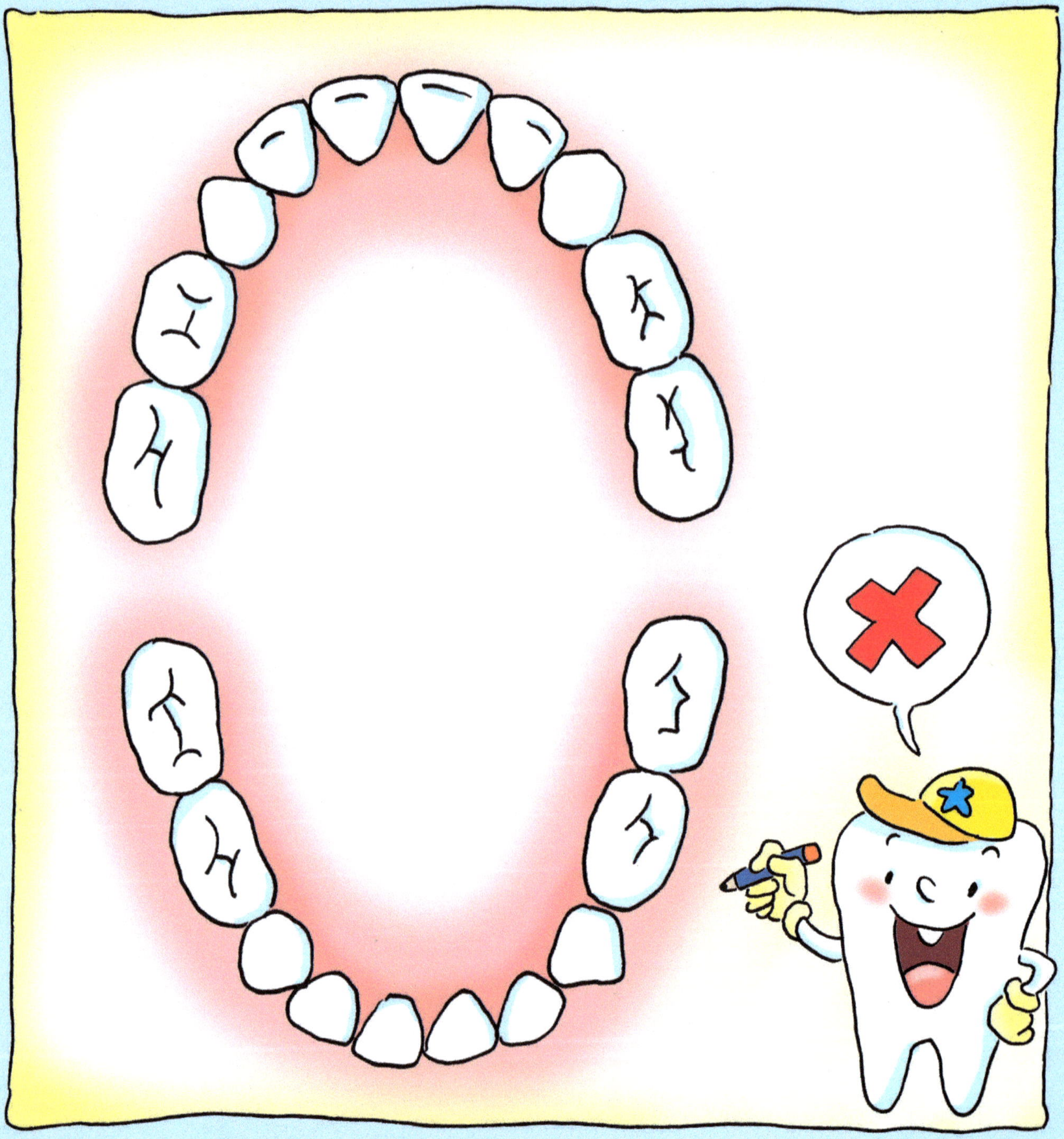

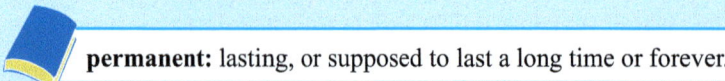

Name: Class: Date:

Lessons 9 & 10

Caring For My Mouth

Gently brush your gums, teeth and tongue in the morning and night. Floss your teeth and rinse your mouth after eating.

Look at the pictures. What should the superfriends do? Put a tick (✓) in the boxes to show healthy habits for mouth care.

1. Haris has had some chips.

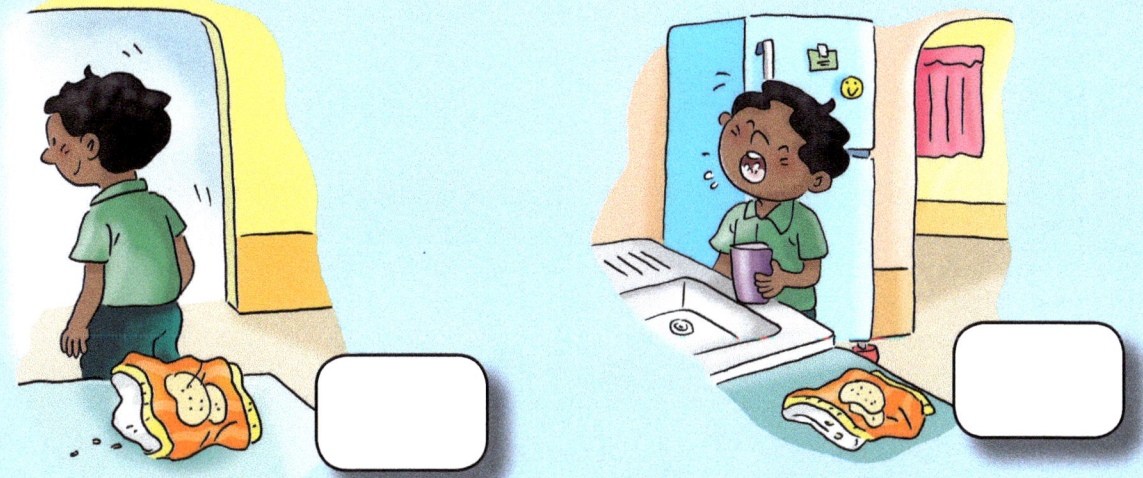

2. Tawan has just got out of bed.

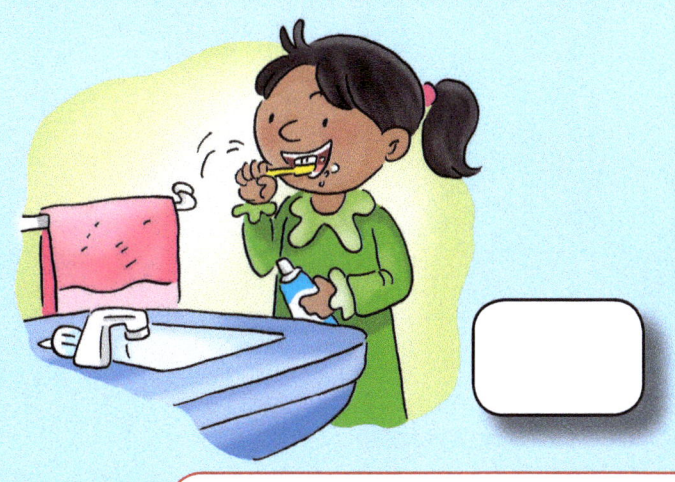
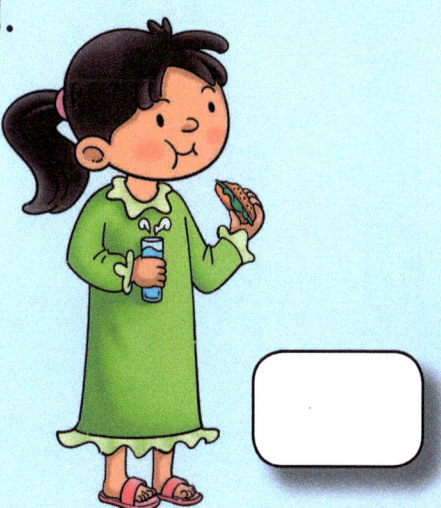

Learning Objective: Pupils will be able to recognise the importance of developing good oral hygiene habits to ensure that the teeth are healthy and well maintained.

3 Eileen has just finished her dinner.

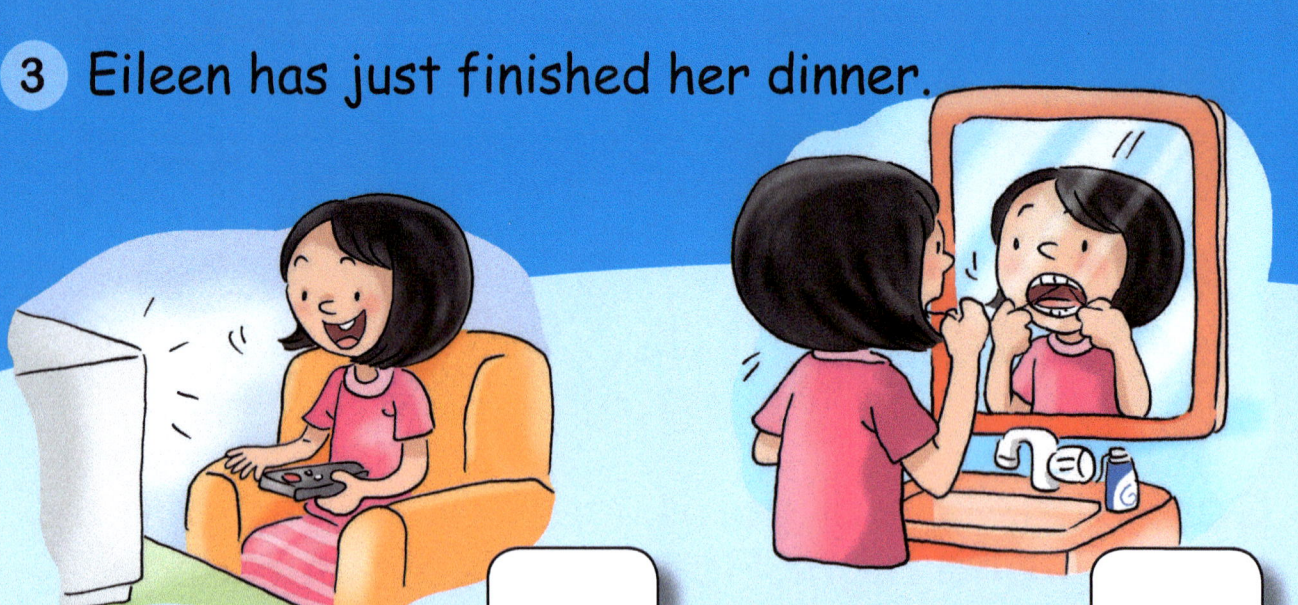

4 Harold has just had some chocolate cake.

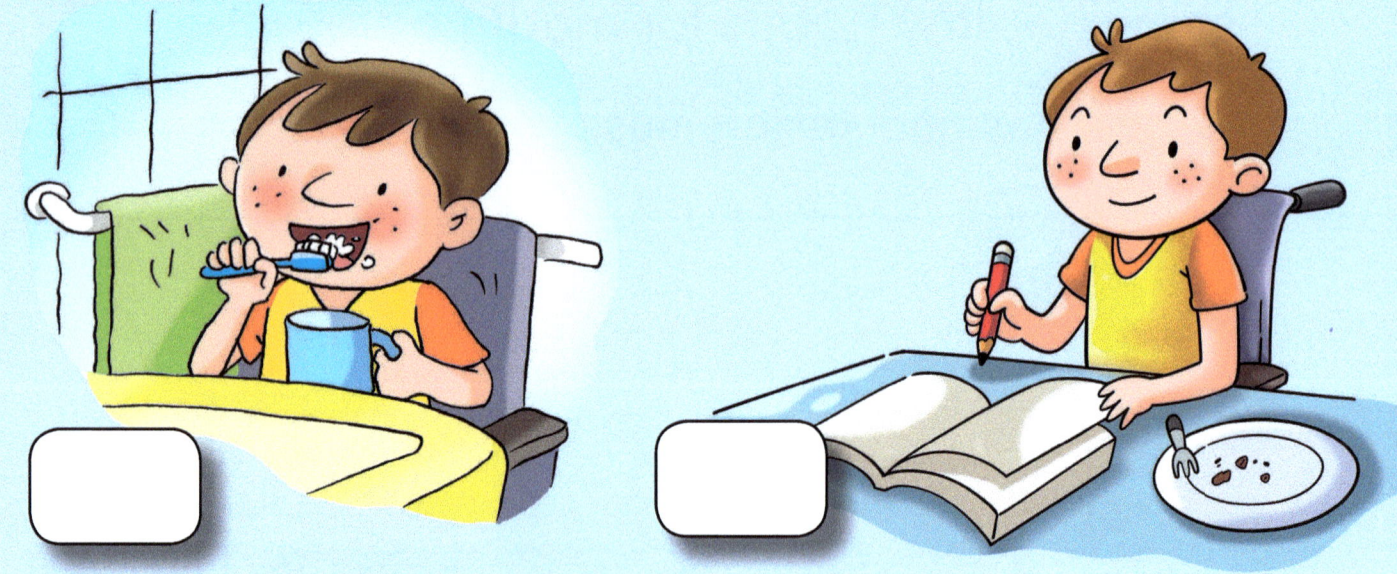

5 Lam is about to go to bed.

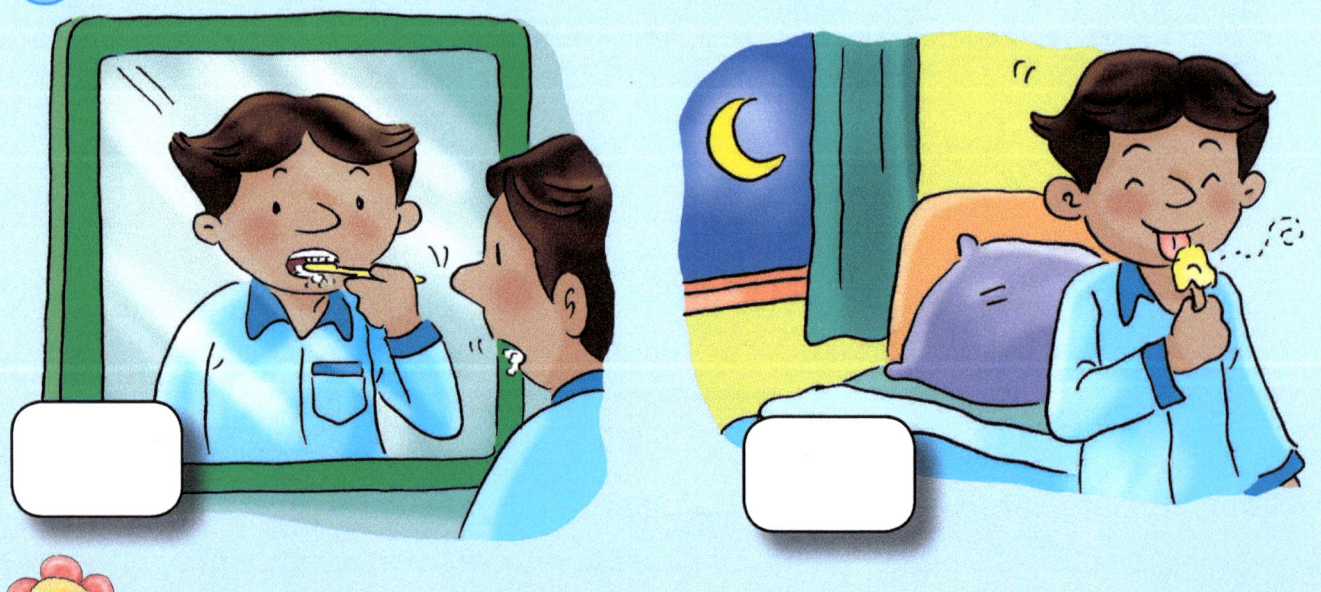

It is important to clean your teeth at least twice a day. When cleaning, first floss your teeth. After flossing, brush your teeth.

1 FLOSSING YOUR TEETH

Ask your parents to choose a dental floss for you.

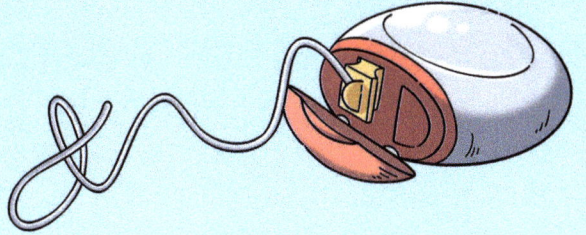

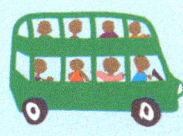
Learn how to hold the dental floss and clean the places between your teeth.
Follow your teacher's flossing actions.

1 Wind 20 to 24 cm of floss round your fingers.

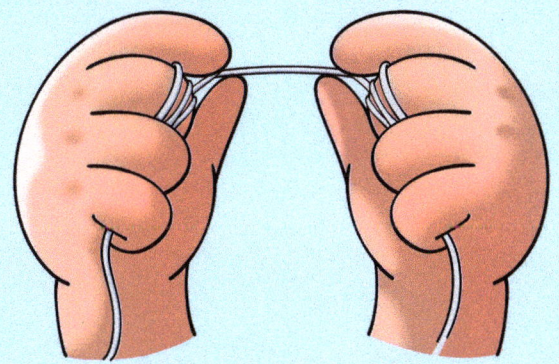

2 Pull about 2 to 4 cm of floss tightly between your two index fingers. Use your thumbs to help you.

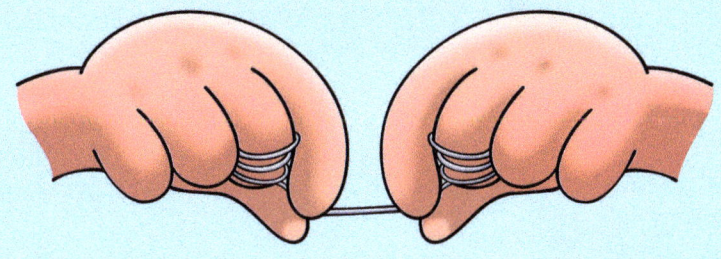

3 Guide the floss between teeth. Gently, clean the sides of the teeth. Floss up and down between teeth.

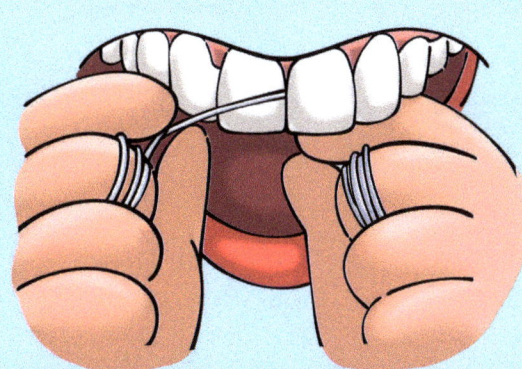

4 Use a clean part of the floss for each space between teeth.

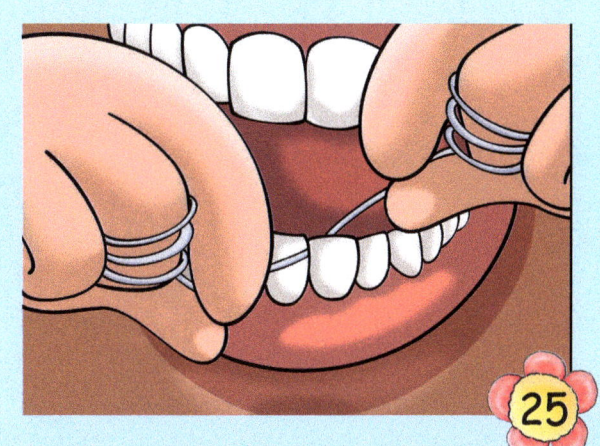

② BRUSHING YOUR TEETH

Choose a toothbrush that is right for you. It should be a soft toothbrush of the correct size. Put a bit of toothpaste on the toothbrush.

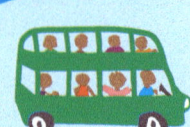 **Learn five different steps when brushing your teeth. Follow your teacher's brushing actions.**

① Place the toothbrush on the outer gums. Brush upwards for the lower teeth and brush downwards for the upper teeth.

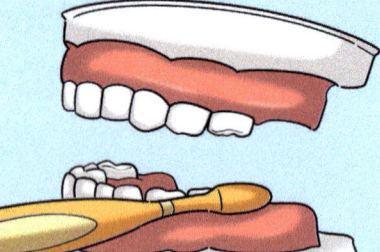

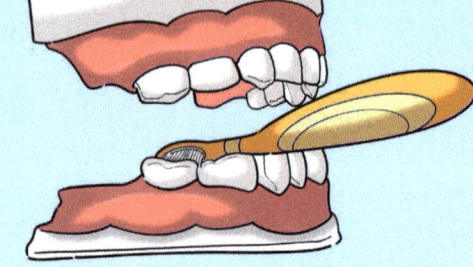

② Brush the inside of your upper and lower teeth.

③ Brush the part of your teeth (the molars) that you use for chewing.

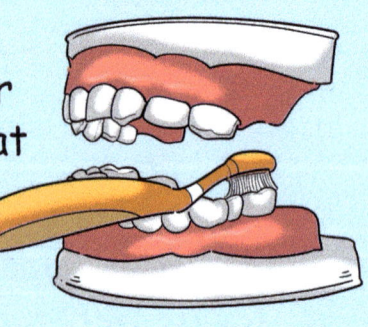

④ Use the tip of the toothbrush and brush behind each front tooth.

⑤ Gently, brush your tongue and gum line.

Environment And Your Health

In this section, you will learn how:

- accidents can happen if you are not careful;
- to prevent accidents; and
- to keep safe at home and outside.

Name: Class: Date: Lesson 1

Watch Out!

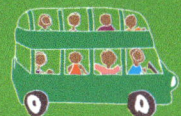 Look at the pictures below. What could go wrong?

1.

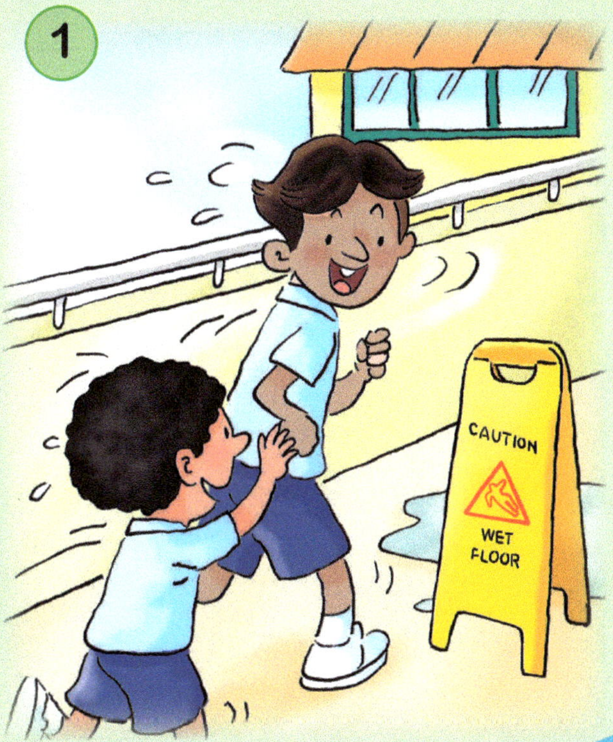

2.

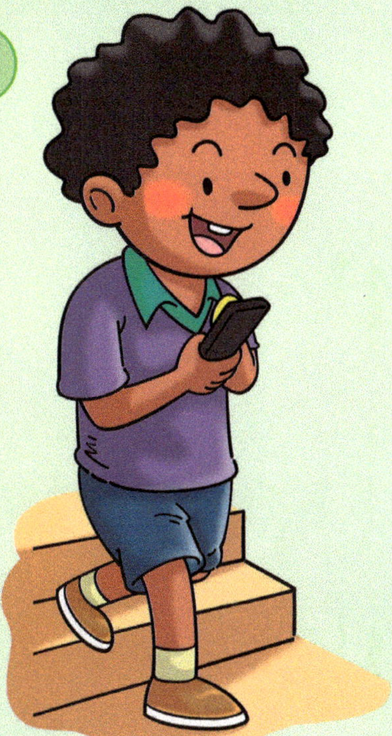

3.

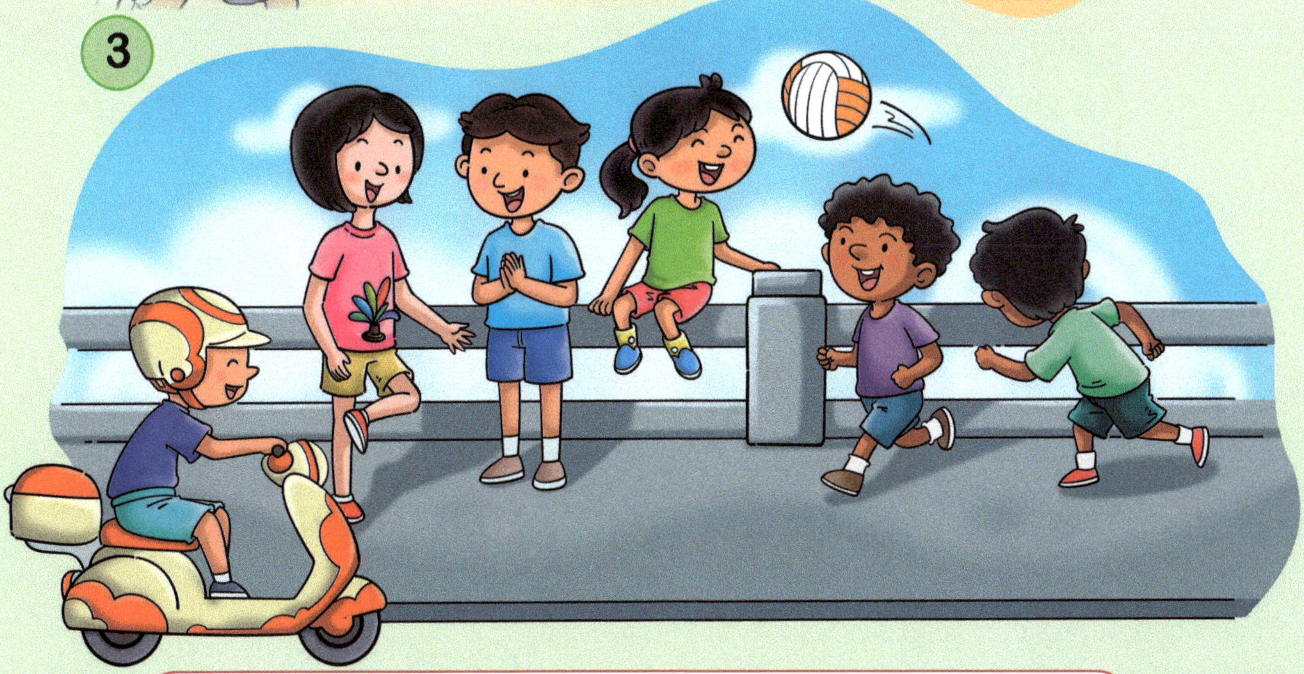

Learning Objectives: Pupils will be able to understand that it is everyone's responsibility to keep safe by paying attention to environmental dangers, and recognise that accidents and unsafe situations can occur in school, at home or in unexpected places and circumstances.

Accidents can happen if you are not careful. You can fall and hurt yourself badly. What should Lam, Tawan, Haris, Ajit and Eileen have done?

Read what they are saying below.

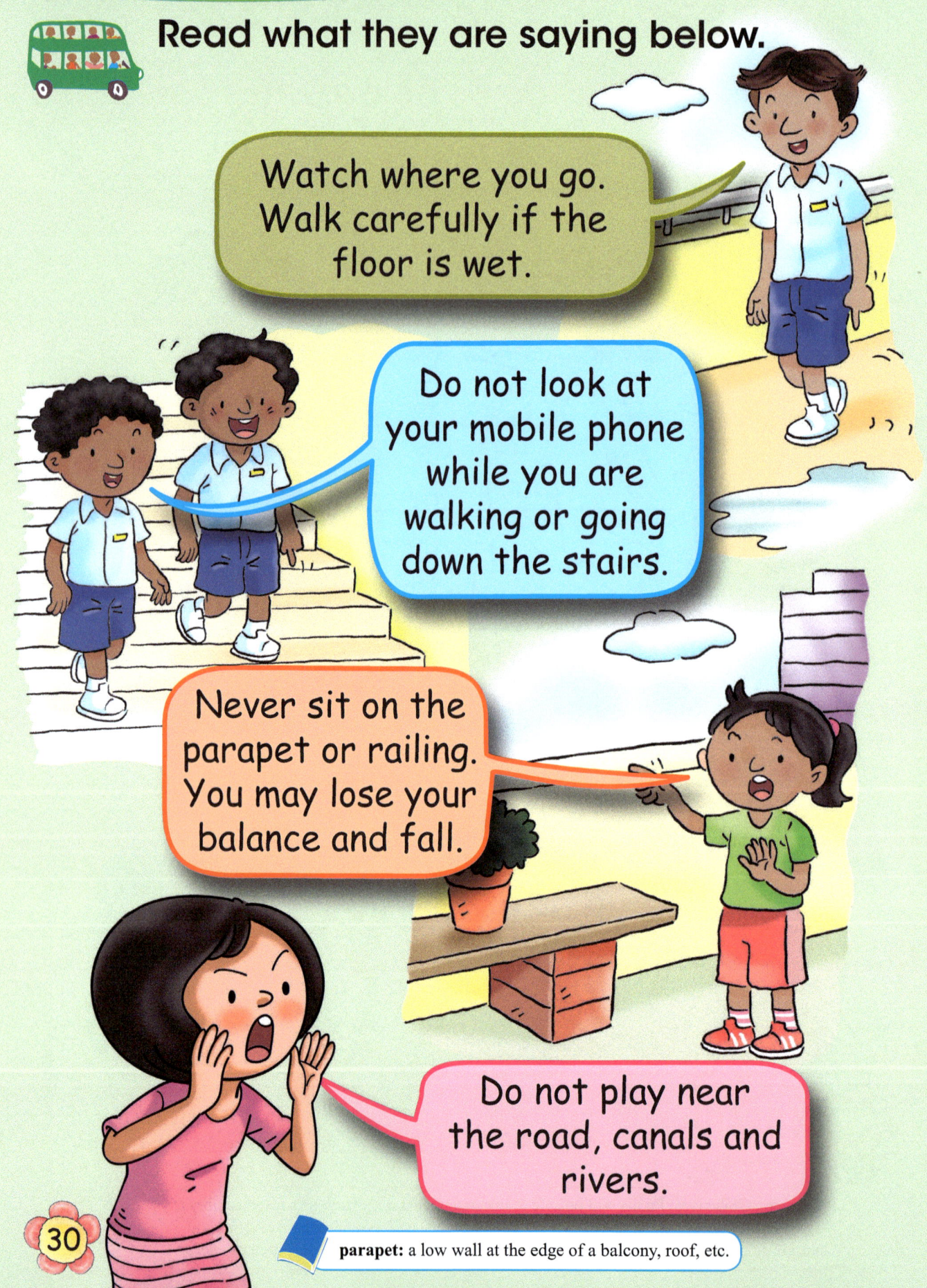

Watch where you go. Walk carefully if the floor is wet.

Do not look at your mobile phone while you are walking or going down the stairs.

Never sit on the parapet or railing. You may lose your balance and fall.

Do not play near the road, canals and rivers.

parapet: a low wall at the edge of a balcony, roof, etc.

Fire, Fire!

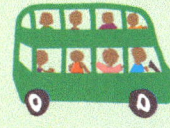 Follow the story in the comic strip below.

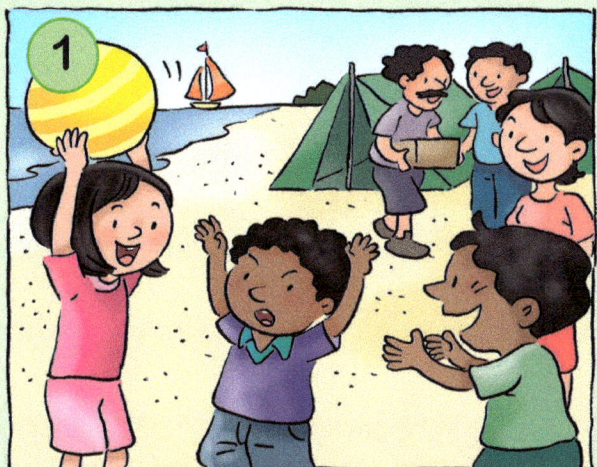

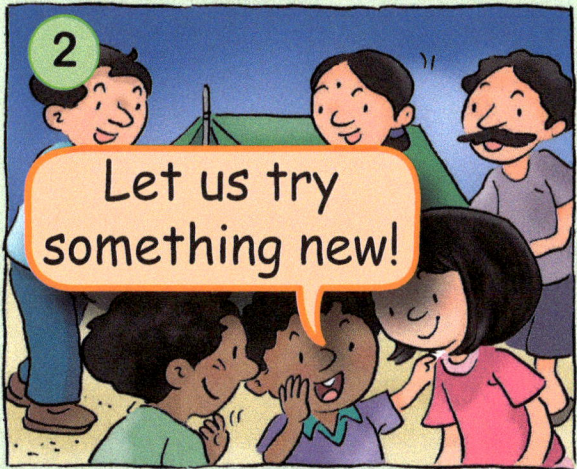

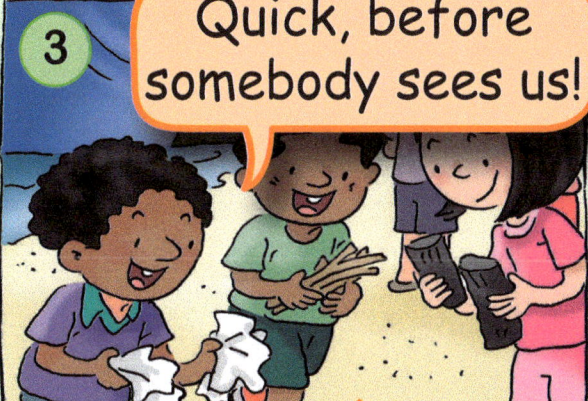

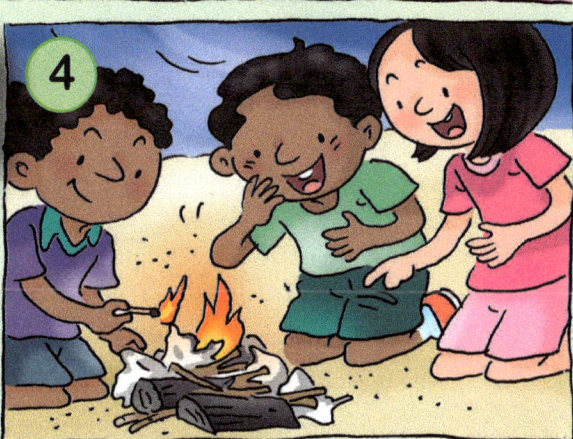

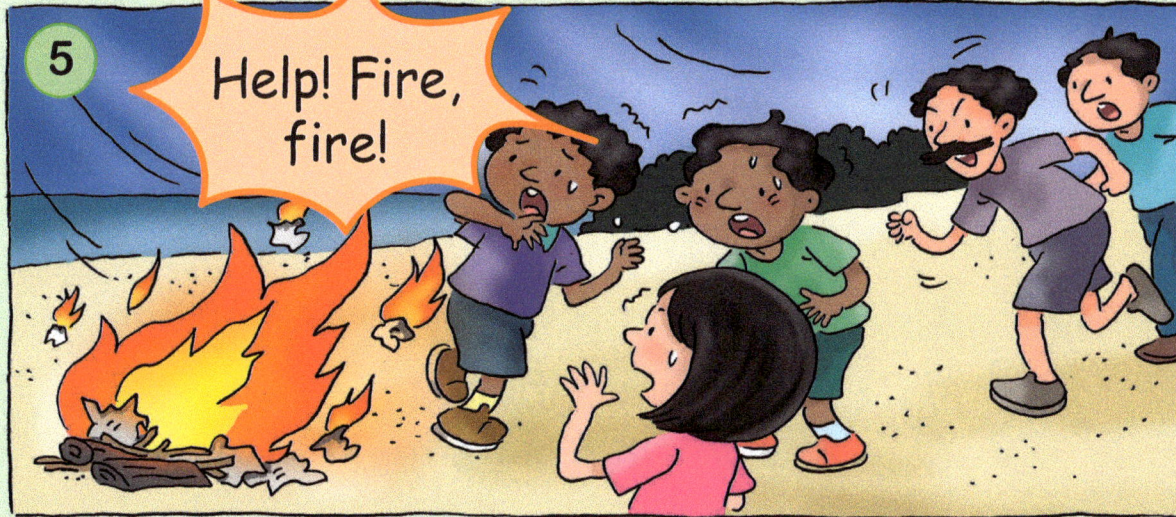

Learning Objectives: Pupils will be able to understand that it is everyone's responsibility to keep safe by paying attention to environmental dangers, and recognise that accidents and unsafe situations can occur in school, at home or in unexpected places and circumstances.

We need fire to help us cook our food and keep us warm. However, fire can also destroy things. That is why we must never play with fire.

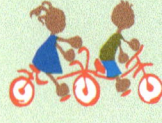 **What will happen if Harold and Lam are not careful? Write your answer in the space below.**

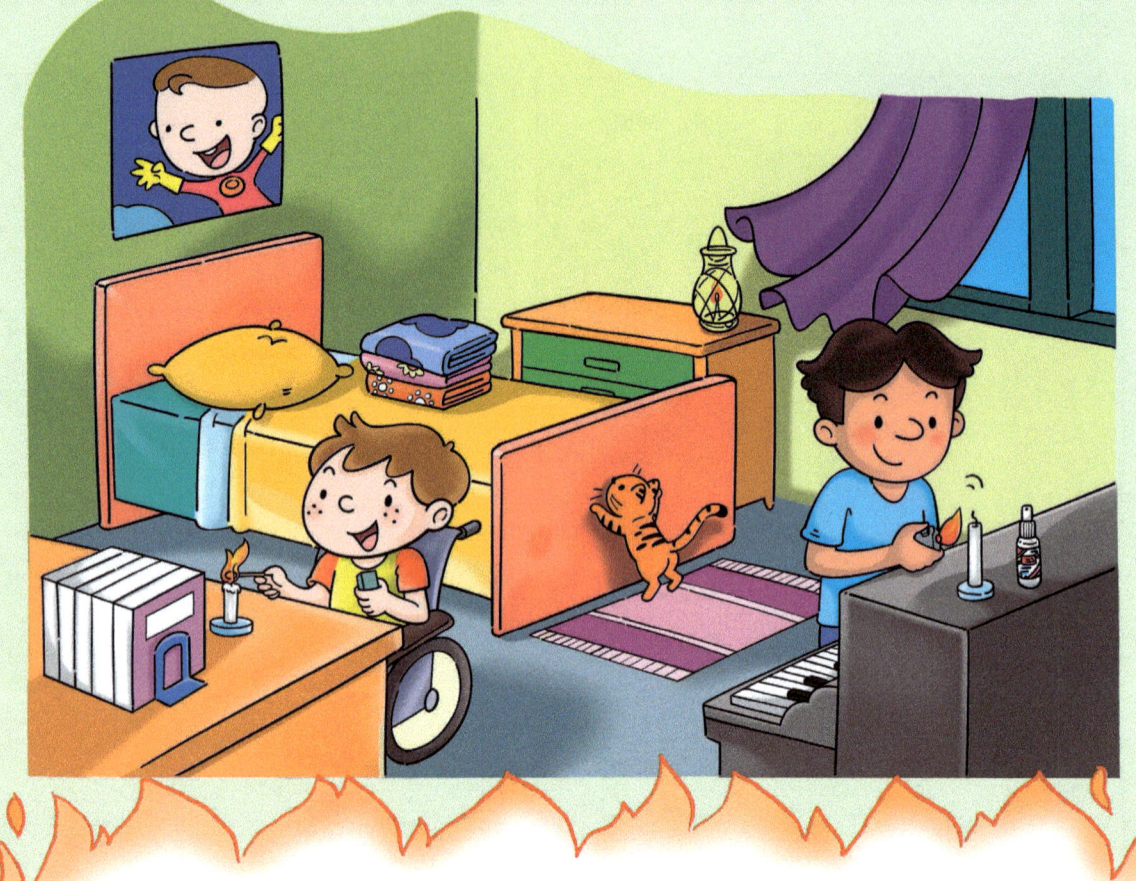

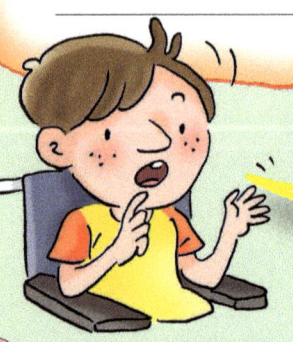 Remember, never play with matches and lighters.

Name: Class: Date:

Lesson 3

Not Water Play

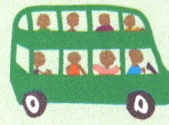 Follow the story in the comic strip below.

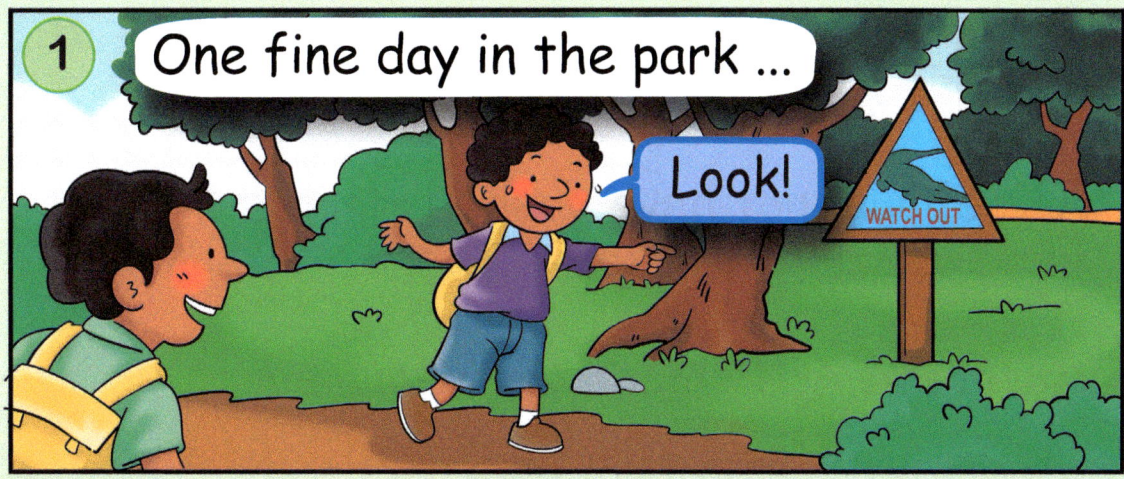

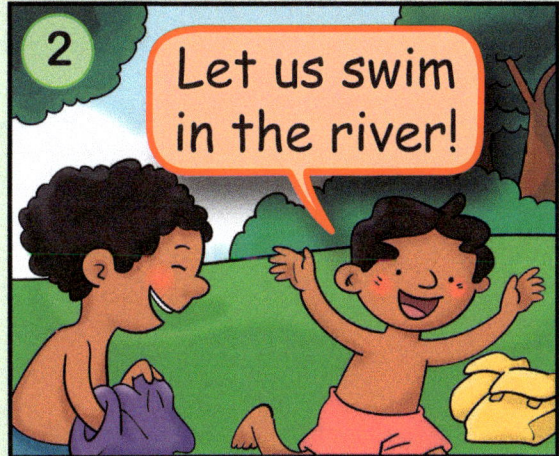
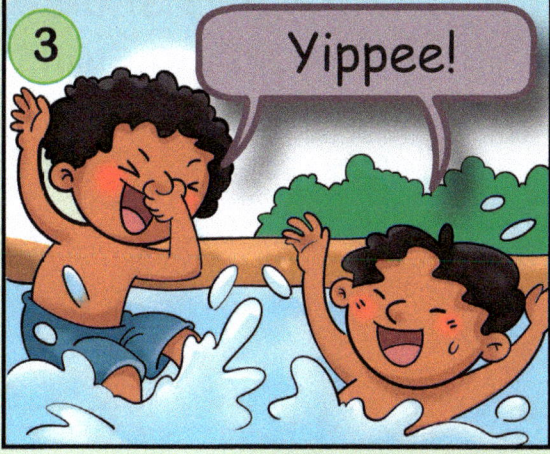

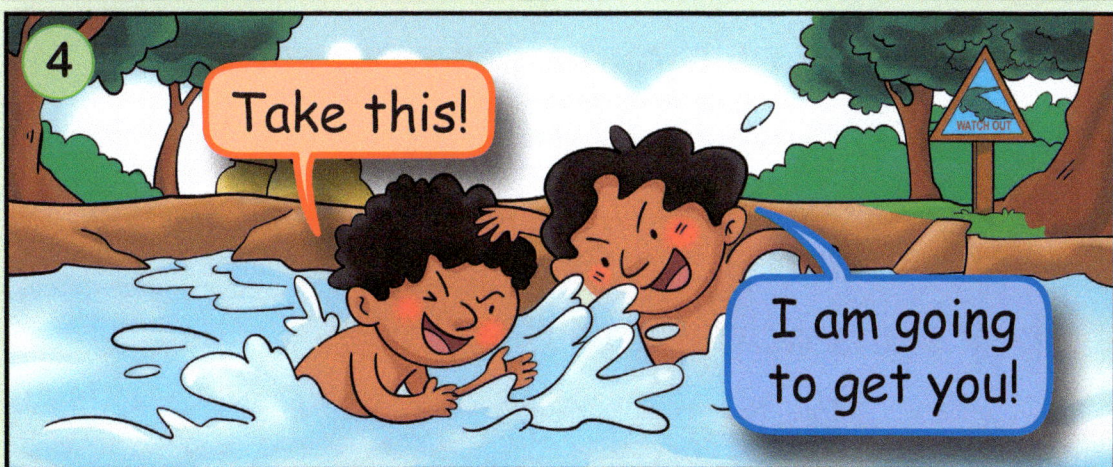

Learning Objectives: Pupils will be able to understand that it is everyone's responsibility to keep safe by paying attention to environmental dangers, and recognise that accidents and unsafe situations can occur in school, at home or in unexpected places and circumstances.

Look at the comic strip again. Read the statements below. Circle 'Y' if your answer is 'Yes' and 'N' if your answer is 'No'.

1. Ajit and Haris did the right thing by jumping into the river for a swim.   Y/N

2. Ajit should have splashed more water in Haris's face.   Y/N

3. Ajit should not have pushed Haris's head under the water.   Y/N

4. Haris and Ajit could have drowned.   Y/N

5. Ajit and Haris should have looked out for warning signs before swimming.   Y/N

You may enjoy swimming, but remember:
- ✔ swim only where you are allowed to do so;
- ✔ always have a parent, guardian or teacher with you; and
- ✔ obey signs warning of danger.

Name: Class: Date:

Lesson 4

Where Do I Cross?

Stay alert to avoid danger. Walk on the pavement.

Circle the superfriends who are crossing the road safely. Put a cross on those who may be in danger.

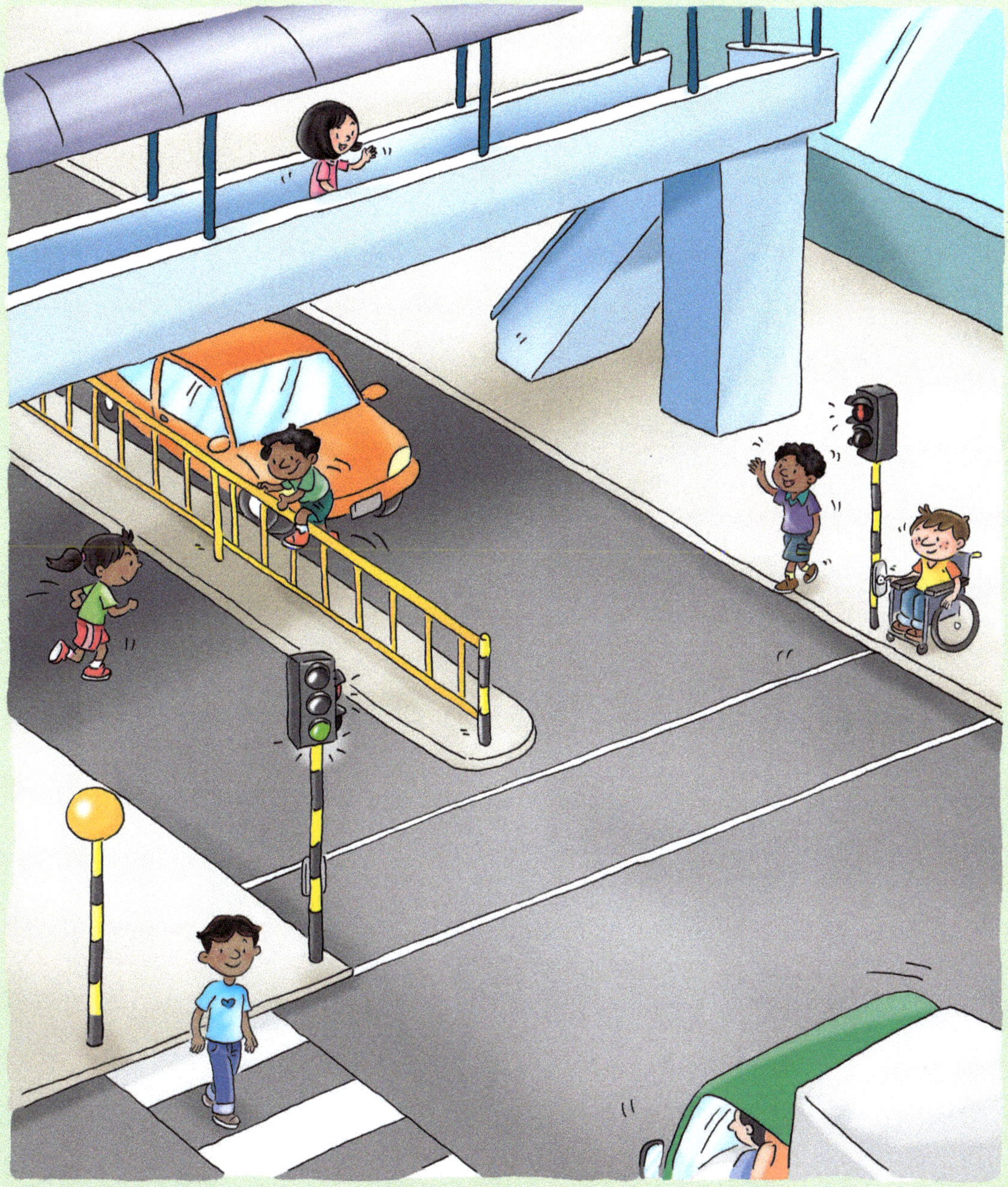

Learning Objectives: Pupils will be able to understand that it is everyone's responsibility to keep safe by paying attention to environmental dangers, and recognise that accidents and unsafe situations can occur in school, at home or in unexpected places and circumstances.

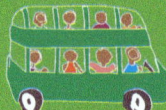

Always use pedestrian crossings when you cross the road.

Overhead bridge
Zebra crossing
Underpass
Traffic lights

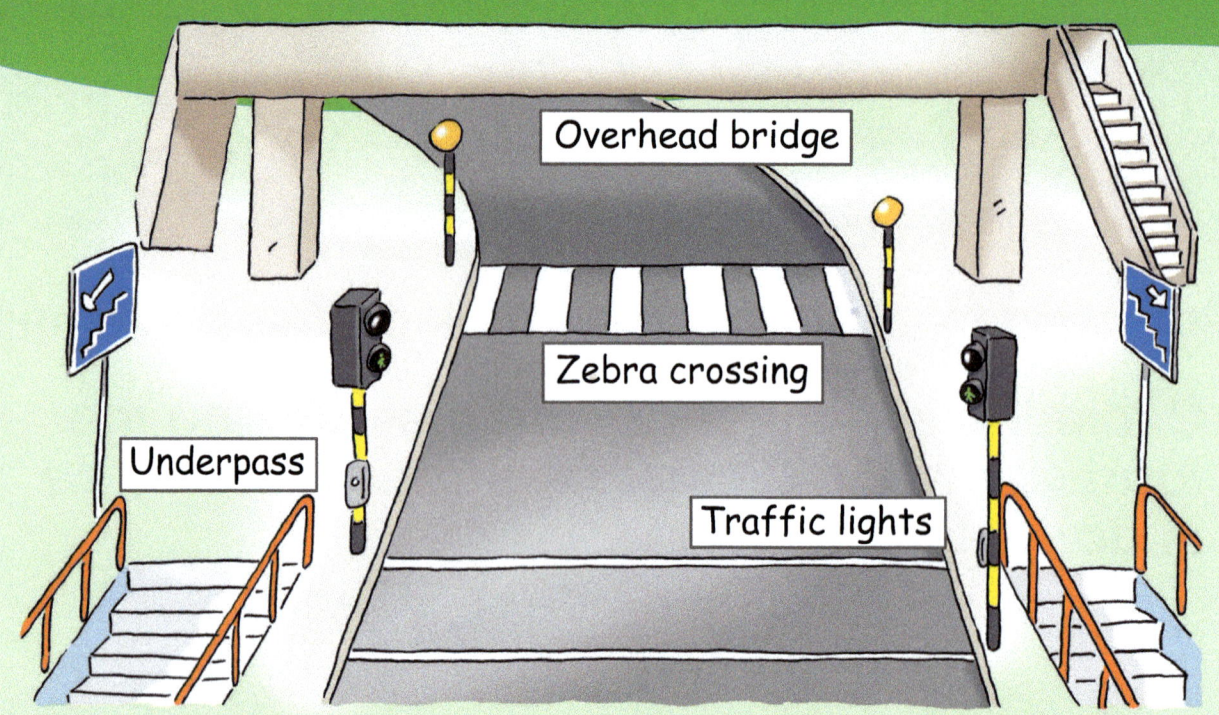

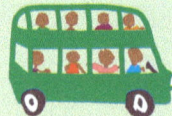

Do the following when you use the traffic lights to cross the road.

1

Press the button to cross.

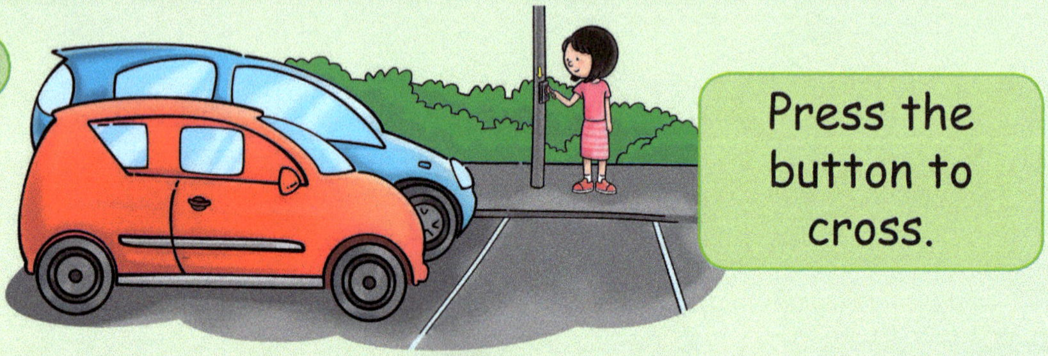

2

Once the light changes, be sure the cars have stopped.

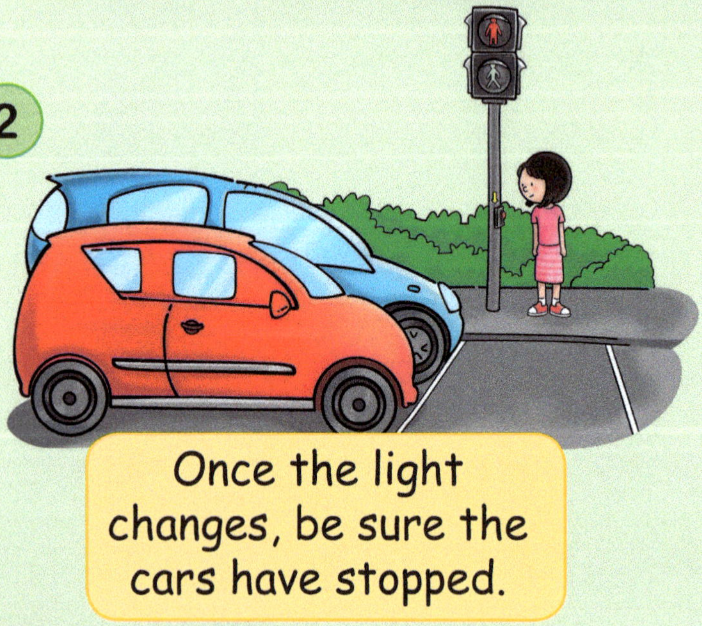

3

Hold up your hand as you cross.

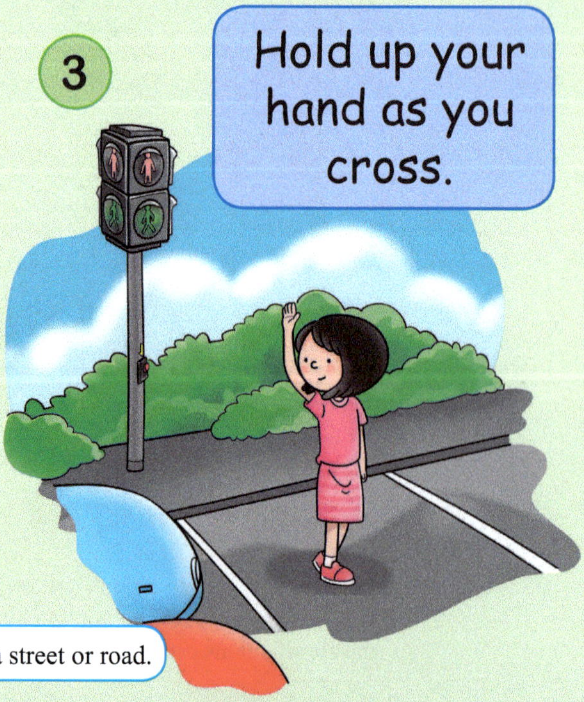

pedestrian: someone who is walking along a street or road.

Name: Class: Date: Lessons 5

Danger!

Look at the pictures below. Which superfriend is doing something unsafe? Put a a cross(✗) in the box next to the picture.

1.

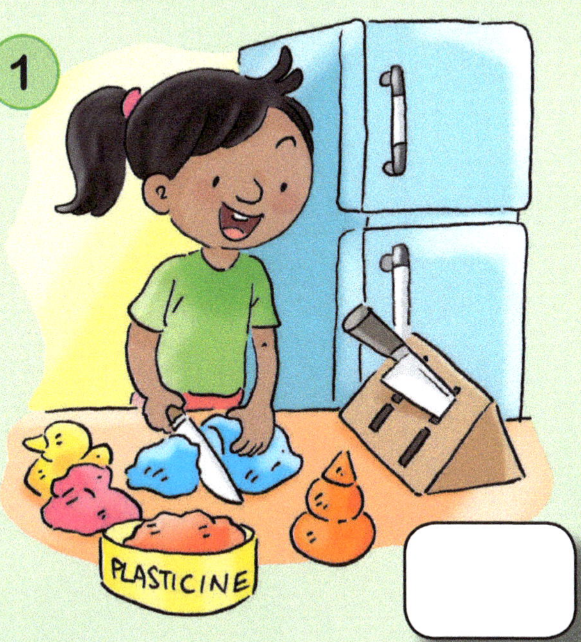

2.

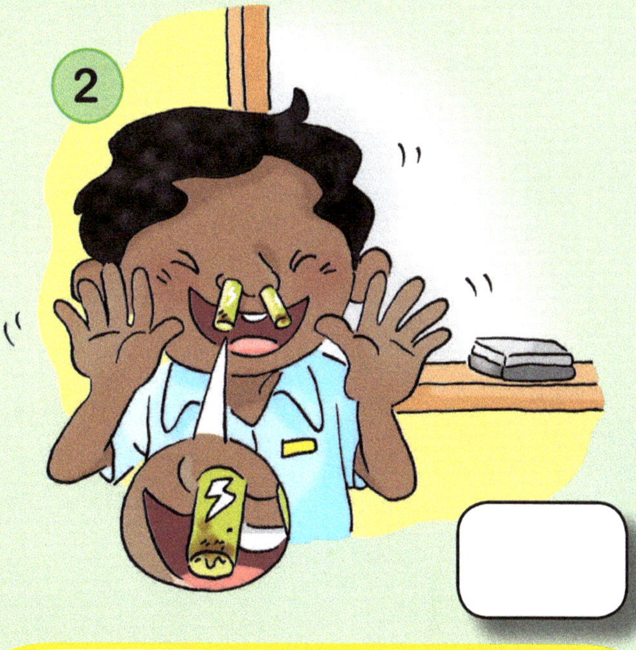

3.

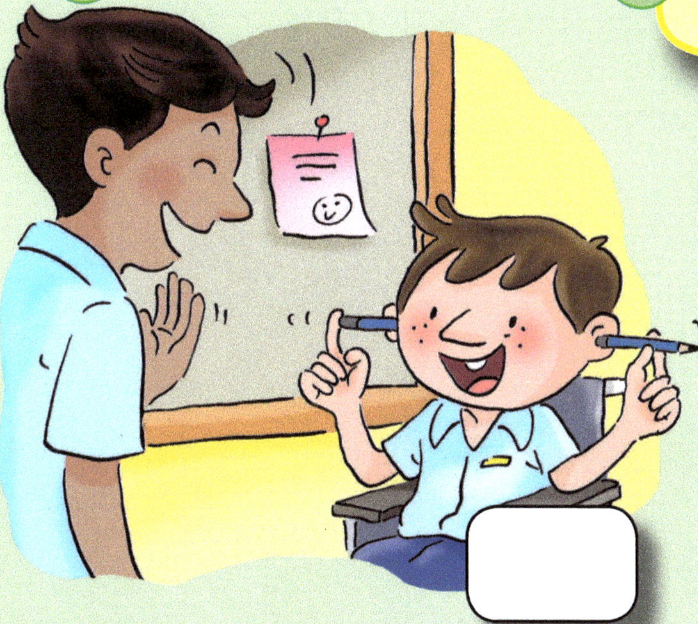

4. Here, take some of this. My mum has a cold too.

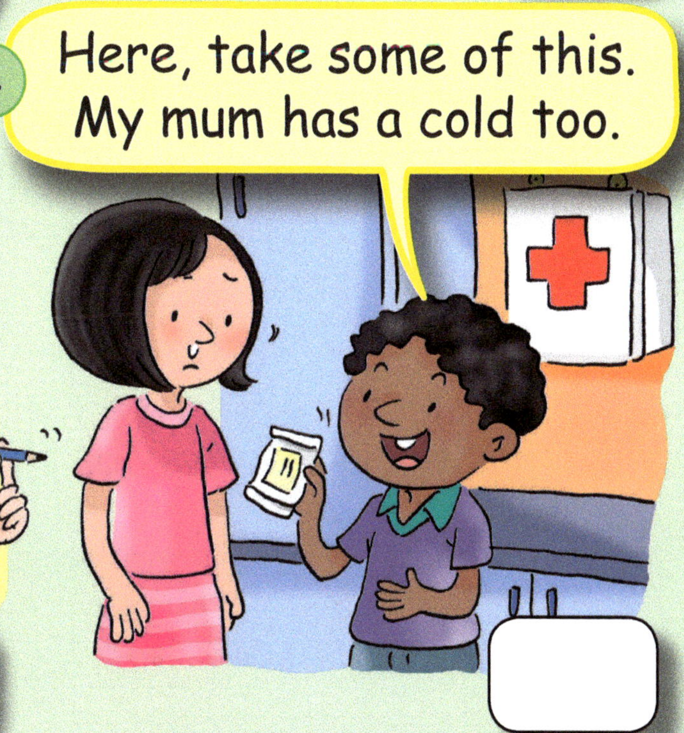

Learning Objectives: Pupils will be able to understand that it is everyone's responsibility to keep safe by paying attention to environmental dangers, and recognise that accidents and unsafe situations can occur in school, at home or in unexpected places and circumstances.

Look at the picture below. Fill in the blanks with the helping words.

lightning	rain	dangerous
thunder	traffic	pedestrian
lighters	toys	vehicles

1. Do not play near the road with your back to oncoming _____ .

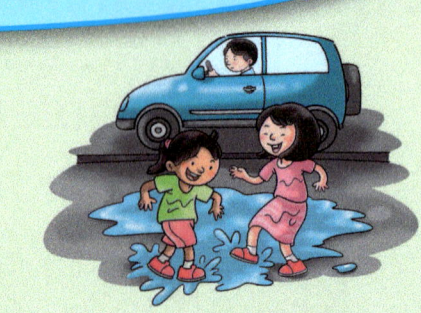

2. Never cross or run across the road when there are no _____ crossings.

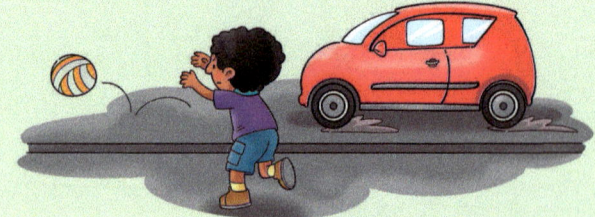

3. Do not play with matches and _____ .

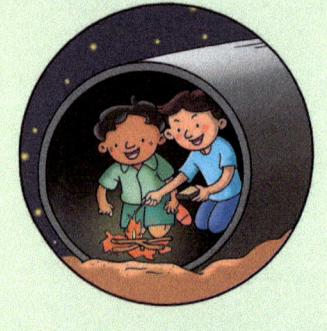

4. Never stand under a tree when there is _____ .

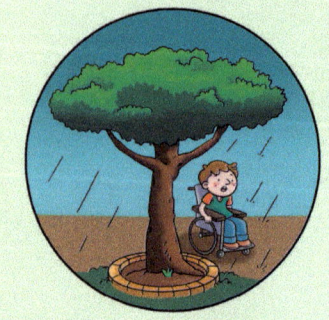

5. Swimming in the river or the sea without adults can be _____ .

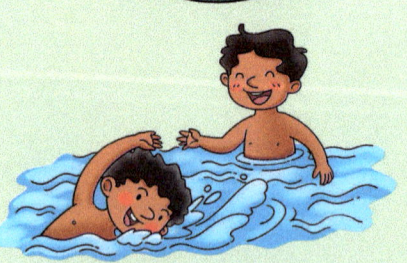

vehicle: a form of transport. Examples include cars, motorcycles, buses, lorries and trains.

Name: Class: Date: Lesson 6

Going Home Alone

Follow the story in the comic strip below.

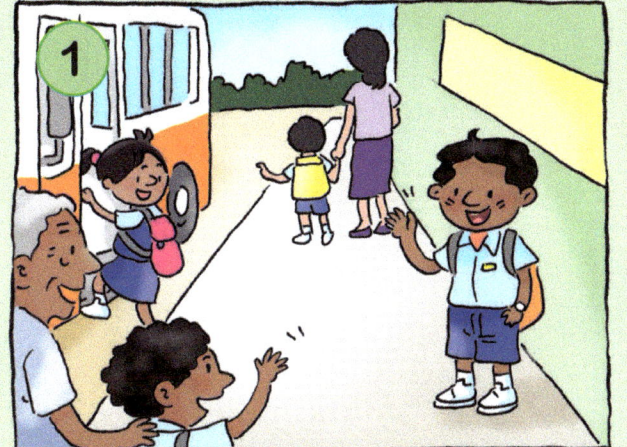
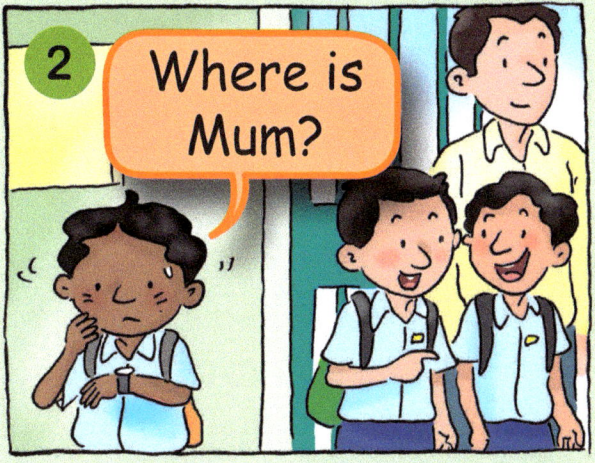
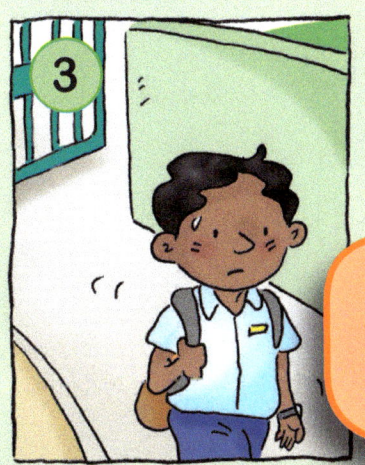
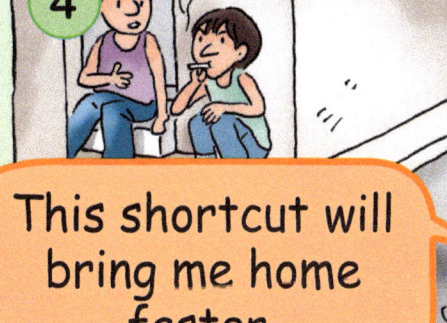
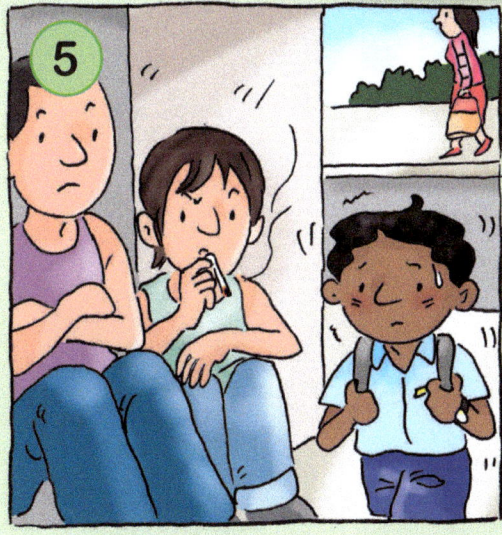
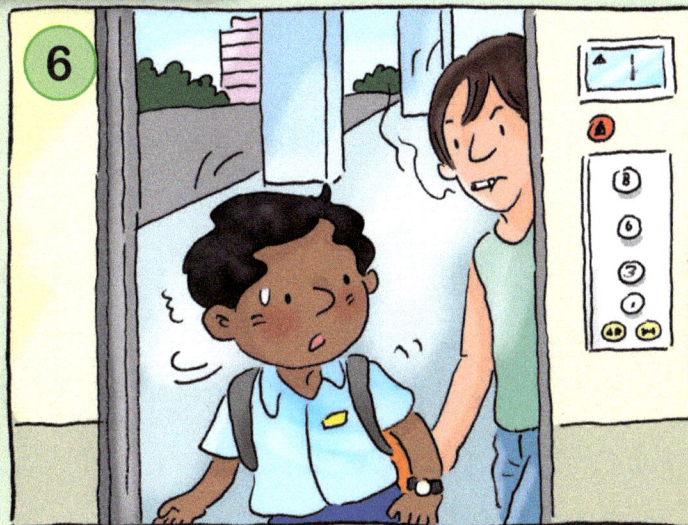

Learning Objectives: Pupils will be able to recognise dangerous situations and react to them in ways to reduce harmful effects.

There are times when you may be alone. You may be waiting for someone or you may be lost. What should you do?

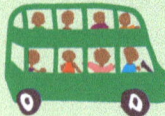 **Look at the pictures and read what Haris says.**

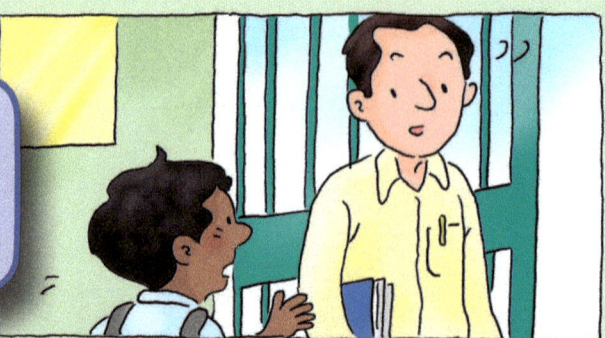

Find an adult you trust to stay with you while you wait.

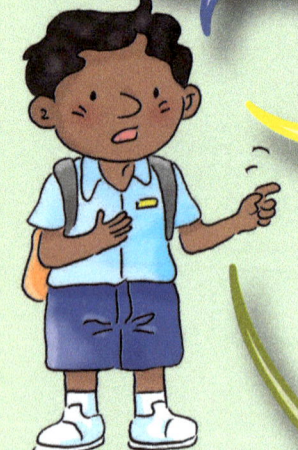

Avoid dark and quiet places.

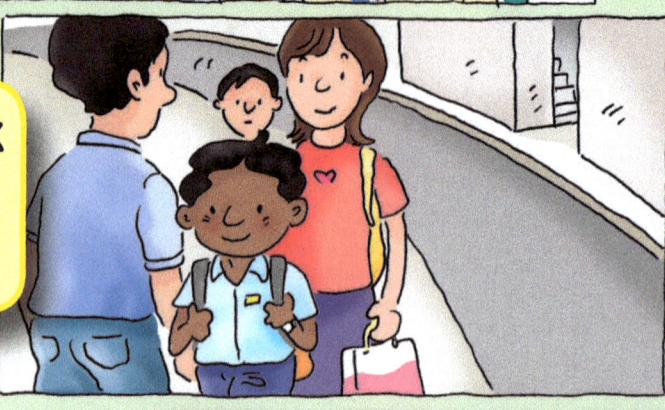

Do not go into a lift with a stranger. Wait for the next round.

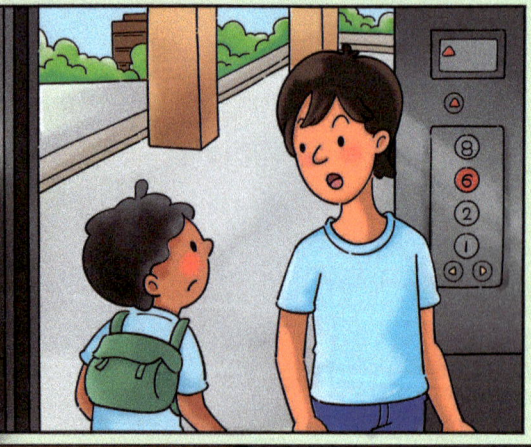

If you need help or feel unsafe, go to your school office or the nearest police station.

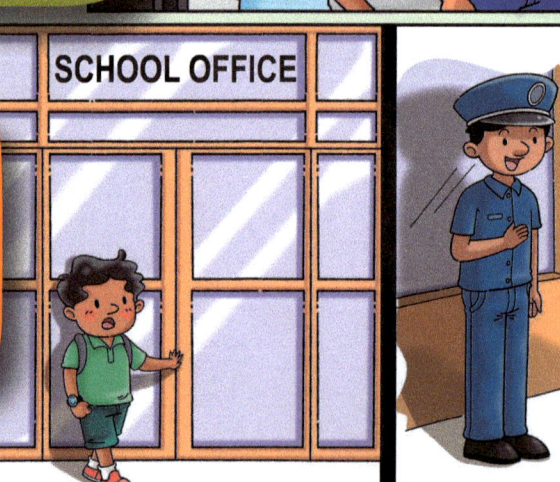

stranger: someone you do not know.

| Name: | Class: | Date: | Lesson 7 |

Be Aware!

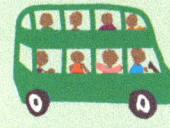 **Look at the pictures below.**

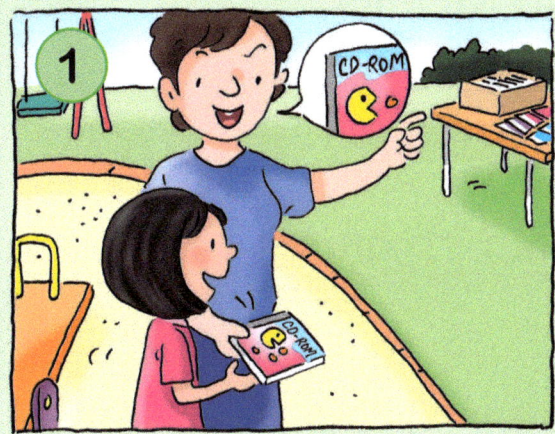
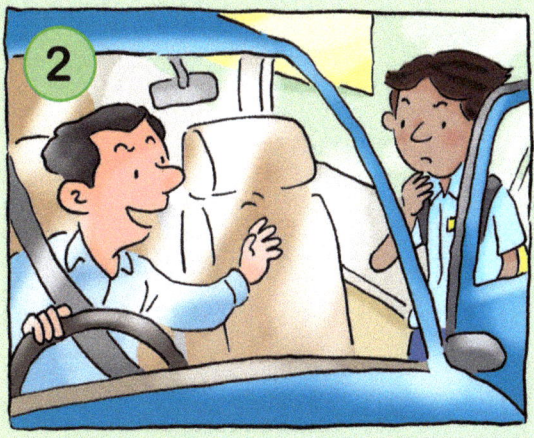
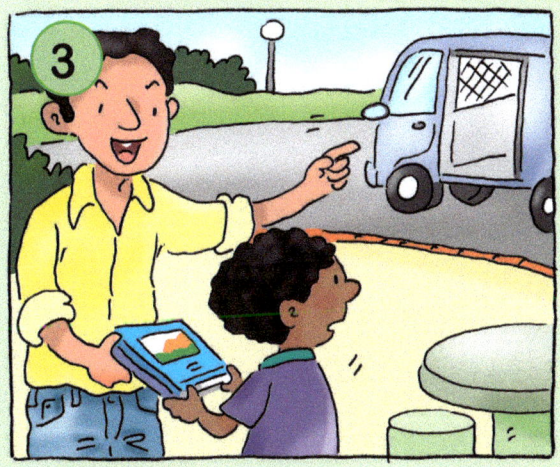
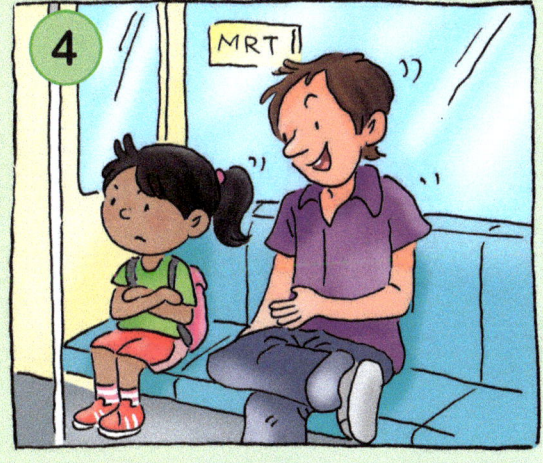
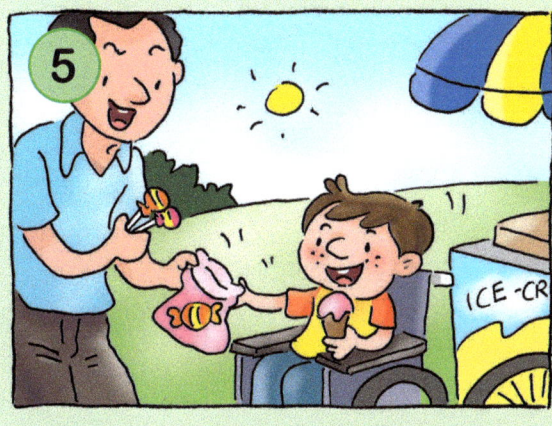
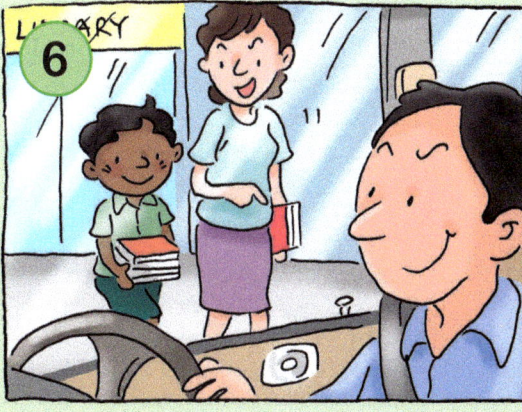

Learning Objectives: Pupils will be able to recognise dangerous situations and react to them in ways to reduce harmful effects.

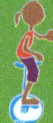

Read the statements below. Circle 'Y' if your answer is 'Yes' and 'N' if your answer is 'No'.

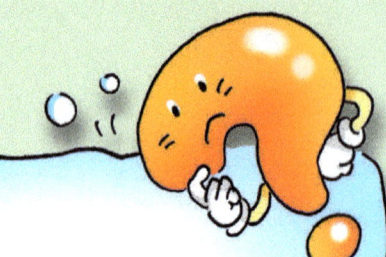

1. I should not accept food, drinks, sweets or cigarettes from a stranger.   Y/N

2. I can accept a gift from a stranger if it is something I like.   Y/N

3. I should accept a ride home from a stranger if that brings me home earlier.   Y/N

4. I should not leave school with anyone I do not know or trust.   Y/N

5. It is all right to talk to strangers because I can make new friends.   Y/N

Always be careful when you are alone and strangers speak to you.
Walk away and tell an adult you know about it.

Name:　　　　　Class:　　　　　Date:

Lesson 8

Should I Go With Them?

🚴 **Listen carefully as your teacher reads. Do you agree with the superfriend's decision? Put a tick (✓) in the boxes if you do and a cross (✗) if you do not.**

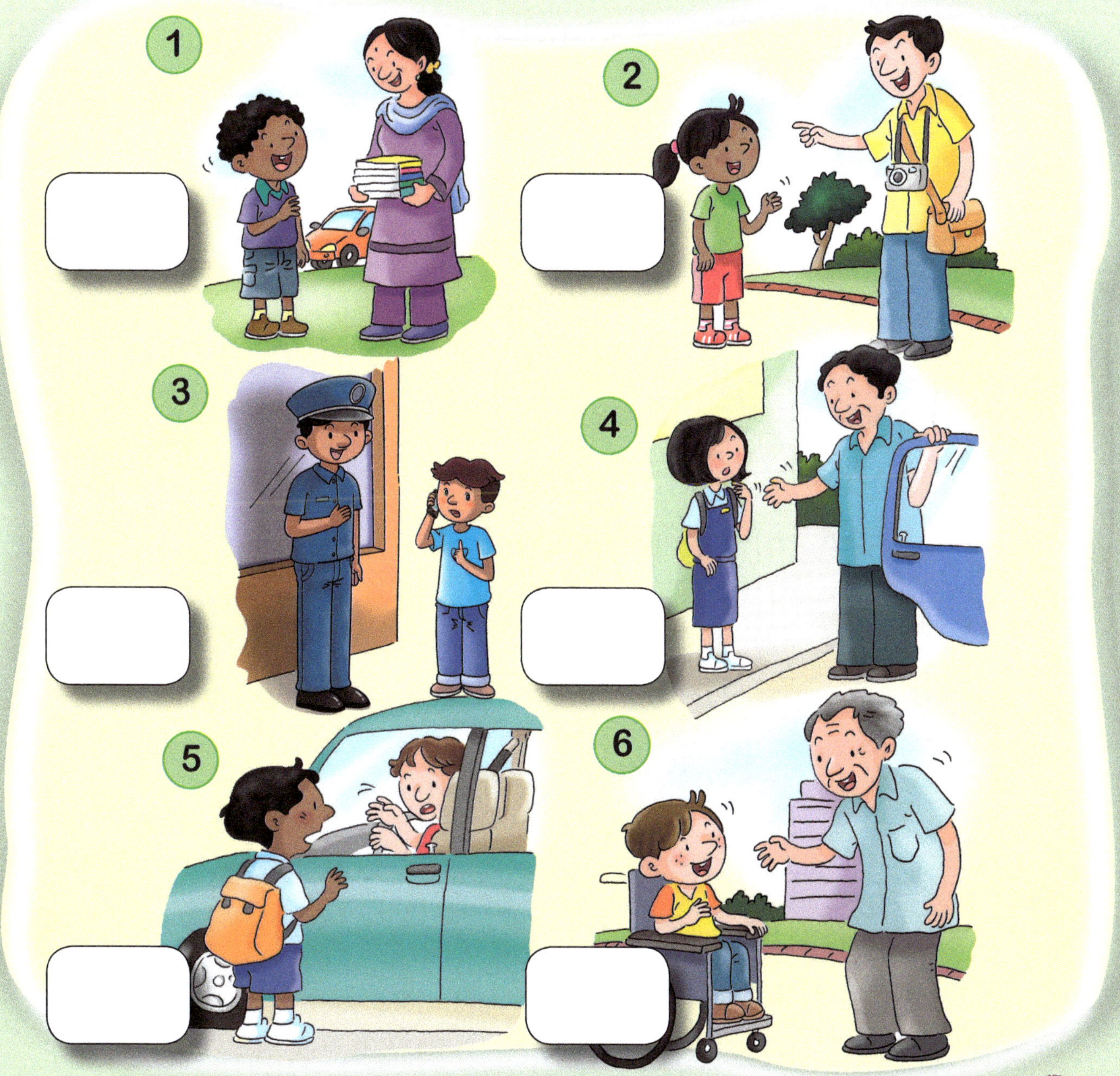

Learning Objective: Pupils will be able to recognise dangerous situations and react to them in ways to reduce any harmful effects.

Not all strangers look scary. Sometimes they are very friendly. People that you do not know very well are considered strangers too.

How can you be safe around strangers? Remember the Safety Pledge.

Safety Pledge

I, _____ promise to check with my parent, guardian or teacher before going anywhere or doing anything with a stranger.

I also promise never to accept things from strangers. I will never help strangers without asking my parent, guardian or teacher for permission.

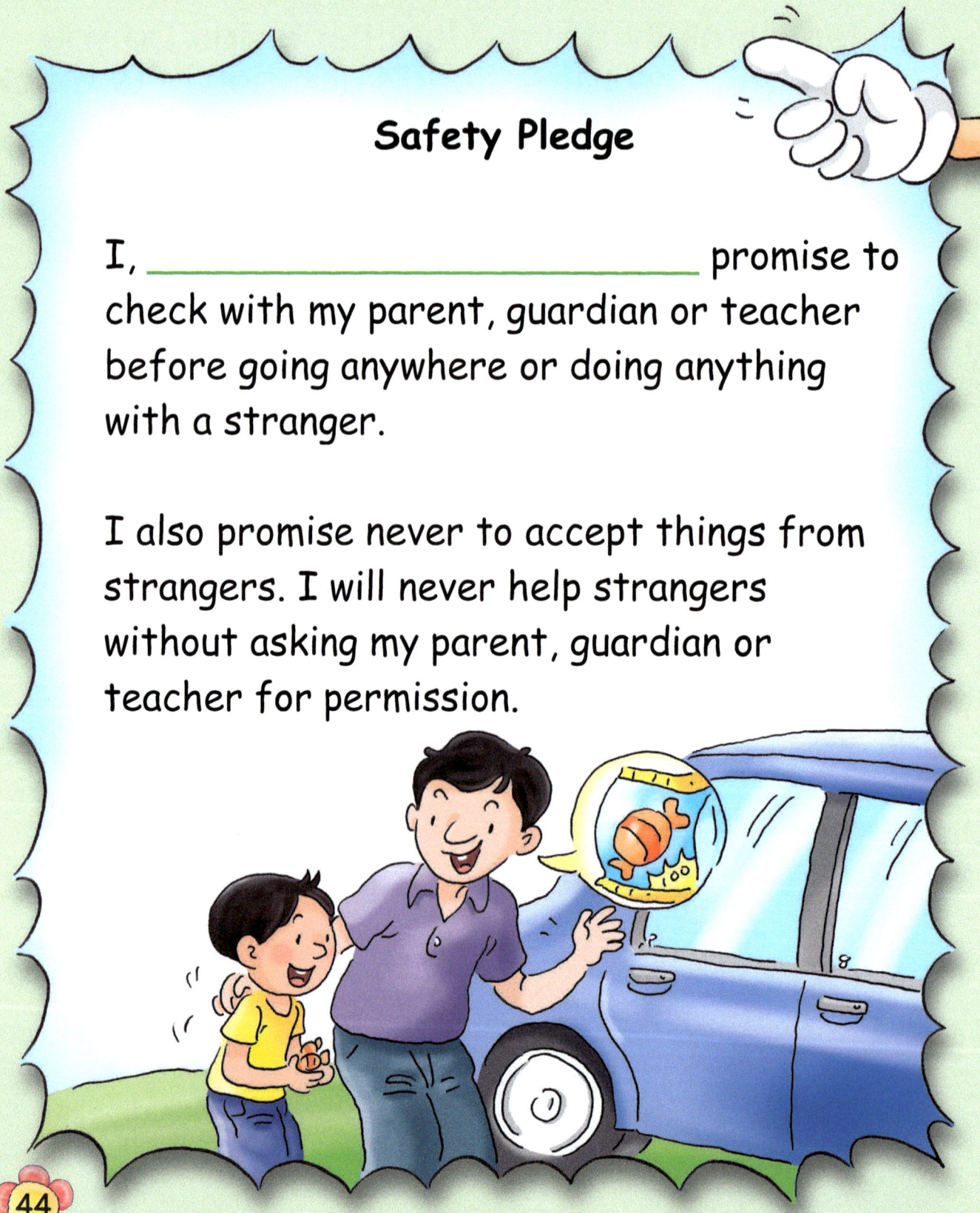

Emotional And Psychological Health

In this section, you will learn about:

- feelings;
- good and unwanted touches; and
- staying safe.

Name: Class: Date: Lesson 1

Feelings

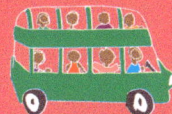 Read the poem.

My Feelings and Me

Sometimes I feel happy,

Sometimes I feel sad.

Sometimes I feel silly,

Sometimes I am scared.

My feelings may change,

They are not always the same,

But I am who I am, you see,

My feelings are only a part of me.

I am so glad to be me,

To be the person I am meant to be!

Learning Objective: Pupils will be able to understand different positive and negative emotions experienced.

47

Everyone has feelings. But not everyone shows their feelings. Even then, feelings shape us and make us who we are.

Look at the faces of the superfriends. How are they feeling?

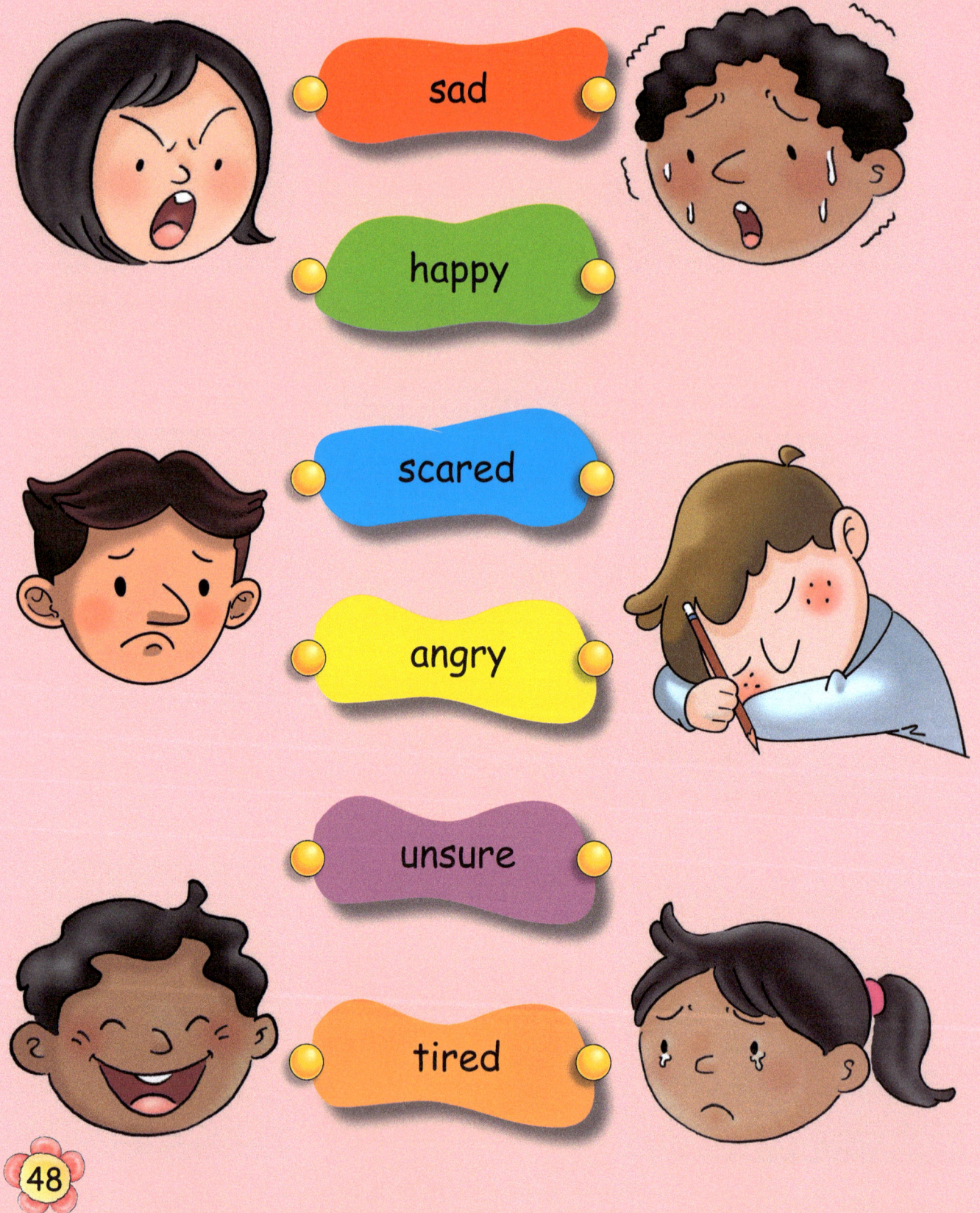

You can have different feelings. Sometimes you can have two or even three different feelings at the same time.

> happy   sad   angry   scared
> excited   surprised   at peace
> relaxed   tired   energetic

How do you feel today? Circle the words above.

Draw a face to show how you usually feel at home and in school.

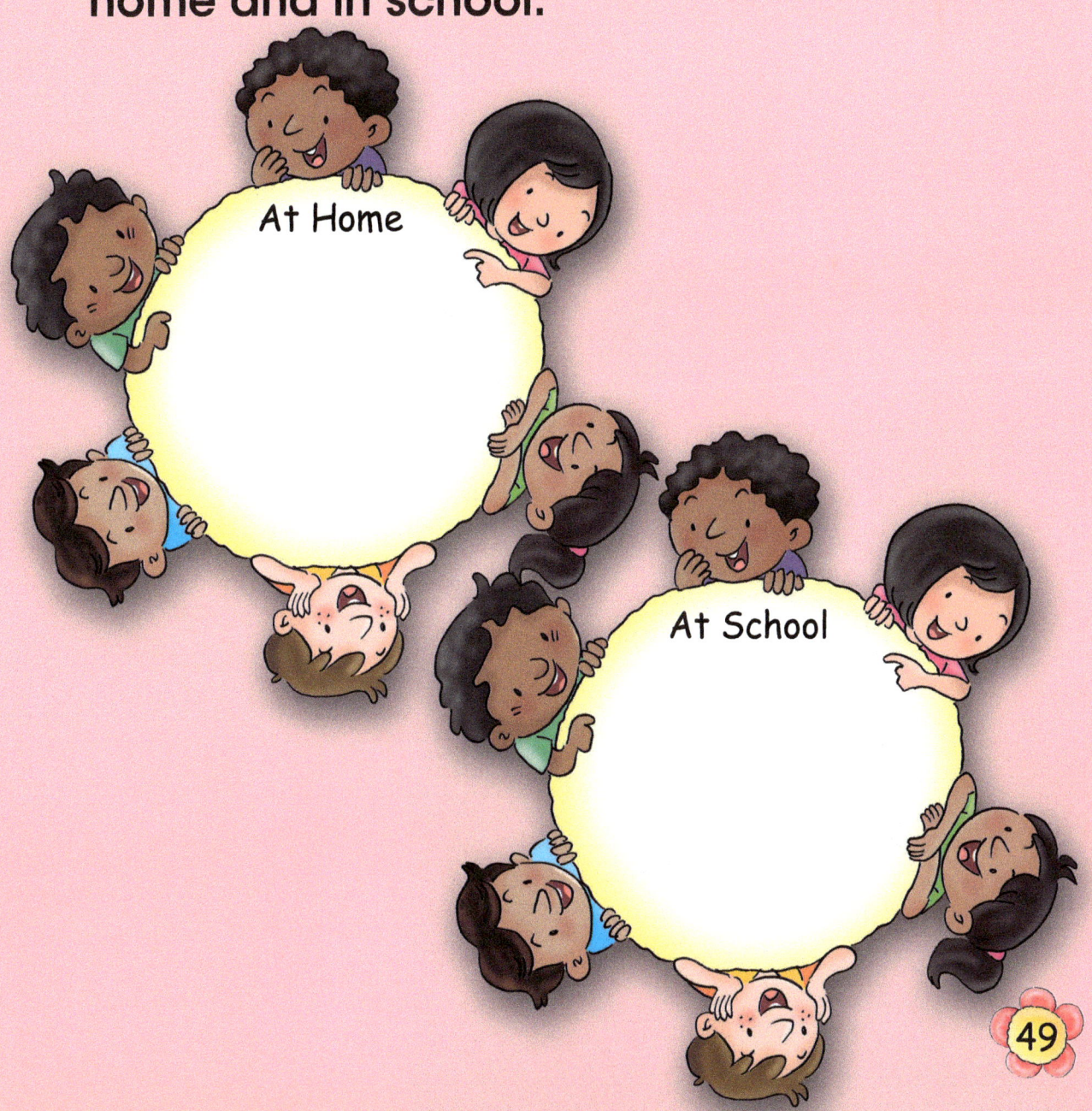

At Home

At School

Let others know how you feel. Trace the leaf below onto a piece of paper. Write your name and how you feel on it. Cut out the leaf and paste it on the Feeling Tree.

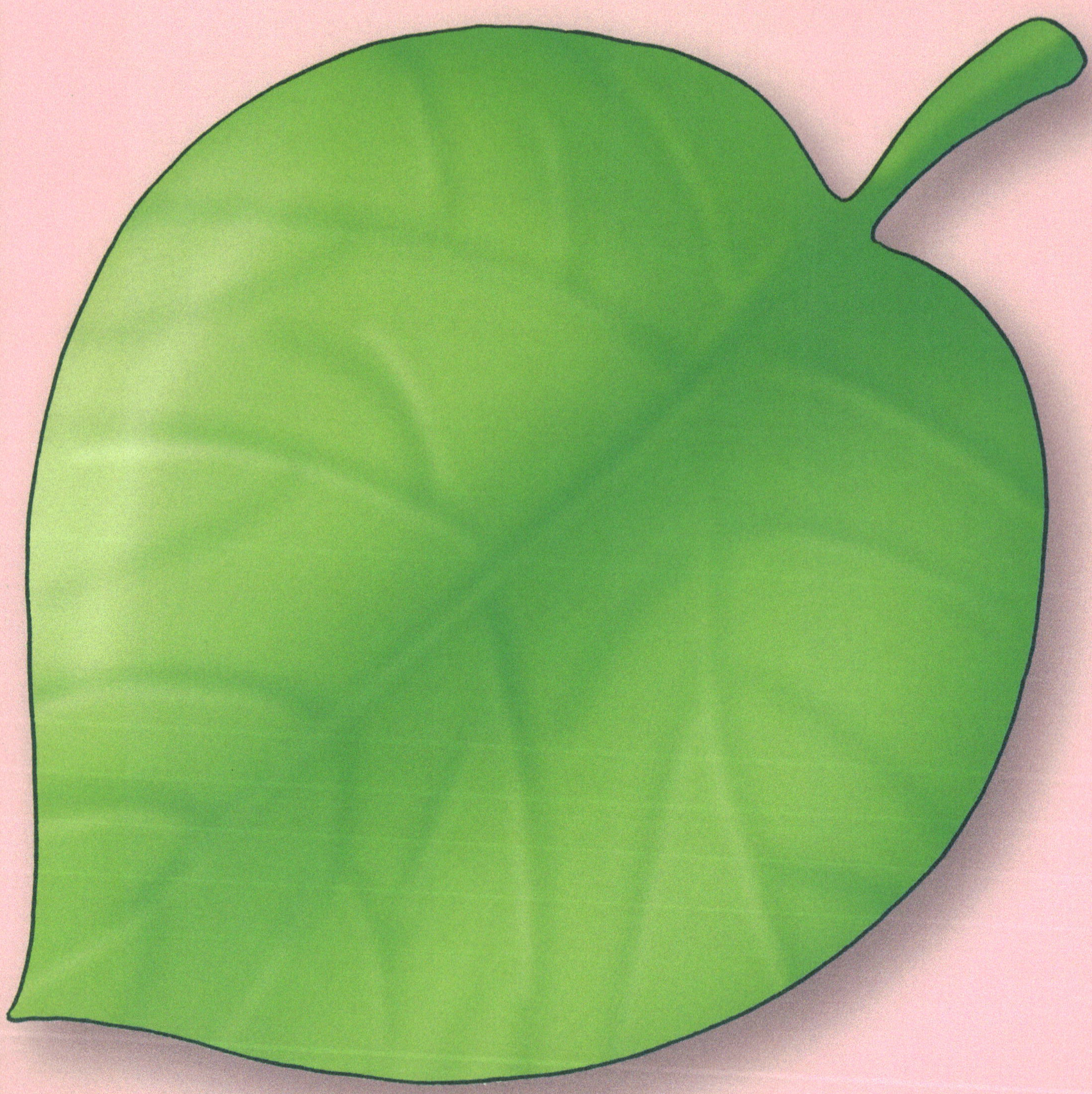

Name: Class: Date: Lesson 2

How Do I Feel?

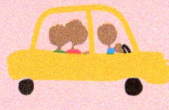 **Look at the pictures. Describe how the superfriends feel.**

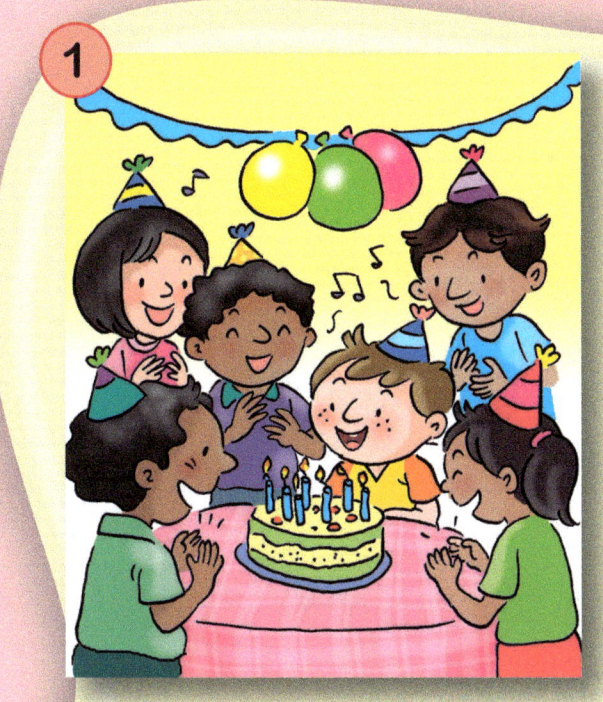

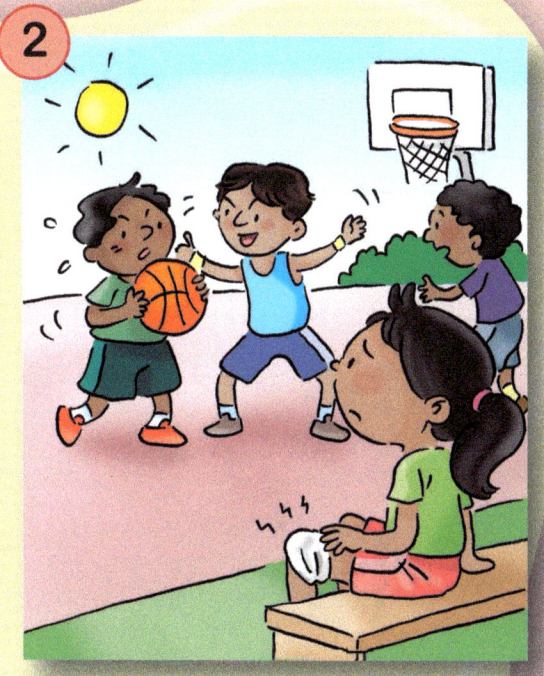

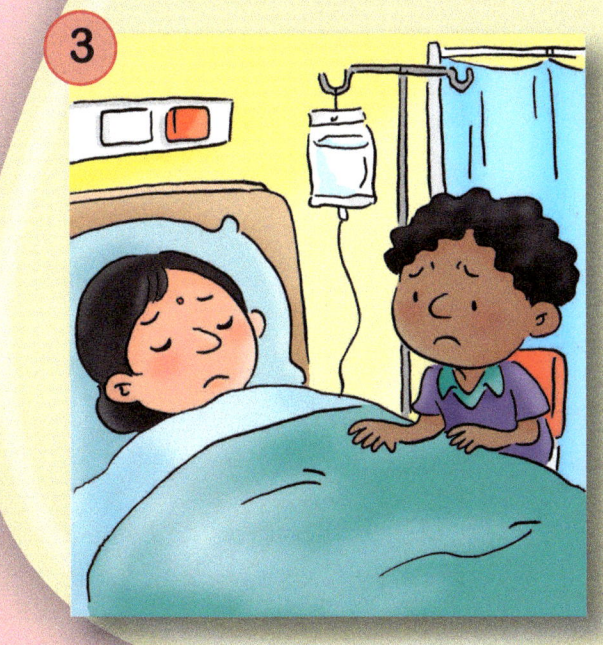

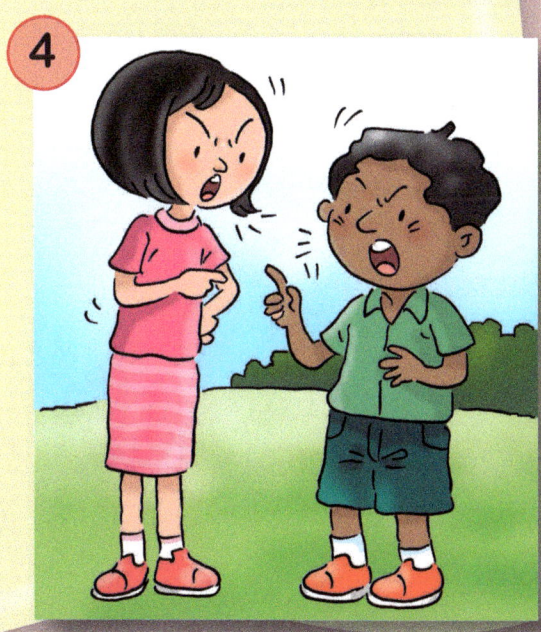

Learning Objective: Pupils will be able to understand different positive and negative emotions experienced.

Sometimes things happen and make us happy. At other times they make us sad, angry or scared.

Imagine you are the pupil in the pictures below. How would you feel? Discuss with a friend. Then draw 😊 ☹️ 😠 or 😨 in the boxes.

happy   sad   angry   scared

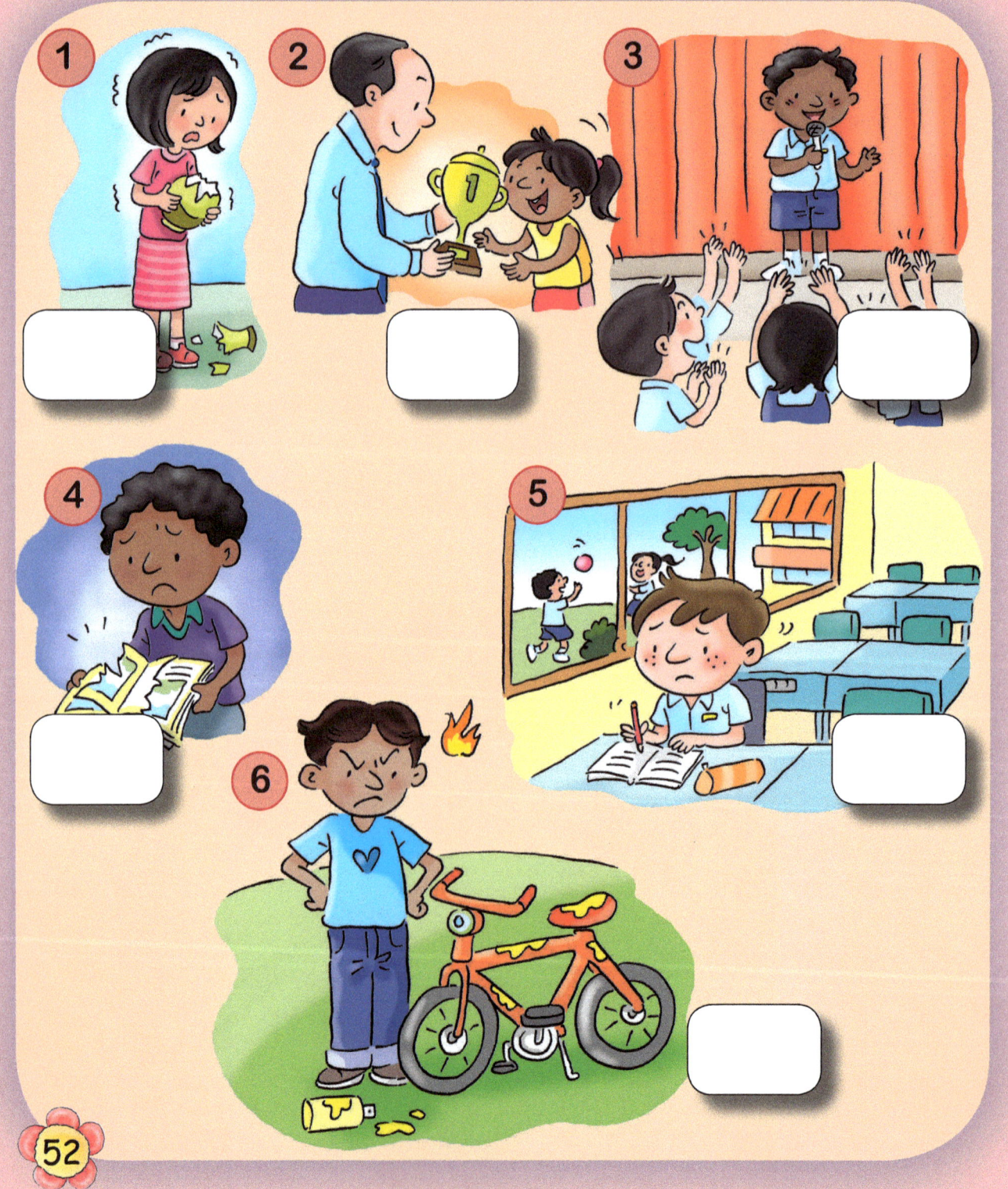

Name: Class: Date:

Lesson 3

In A New Place

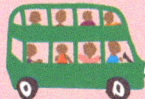 How did you feel on your first day of school? Were you scared, happy or excited? Did you make any friends? Follow the story in the comic strip below.

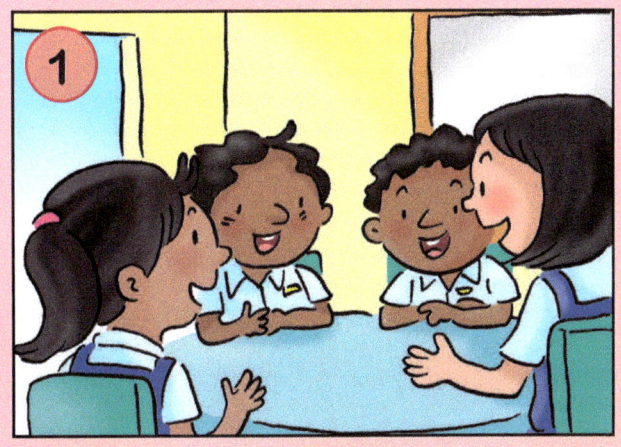
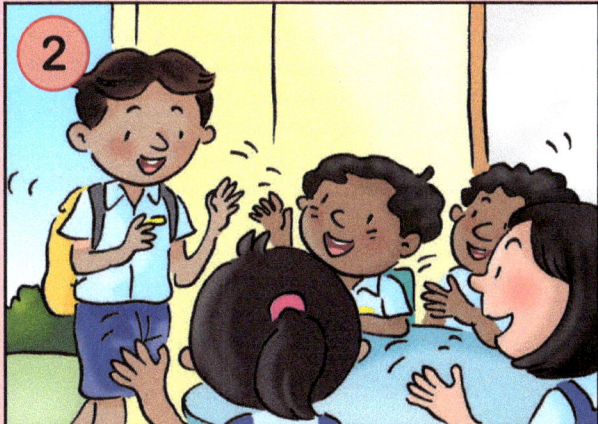
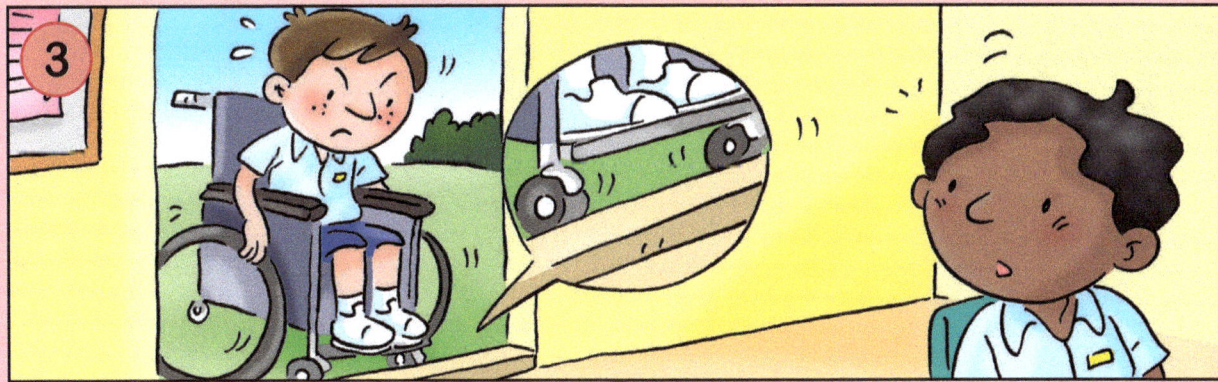
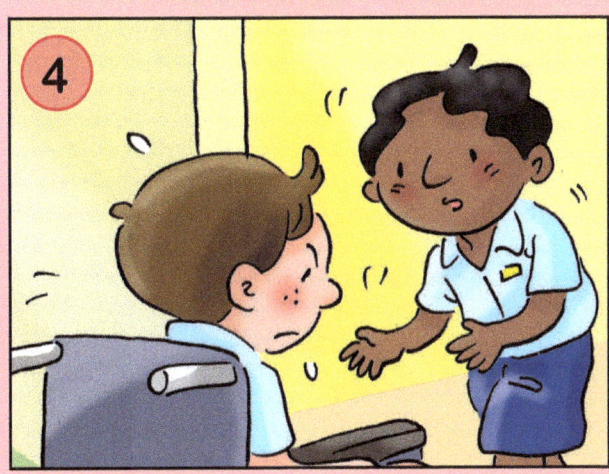
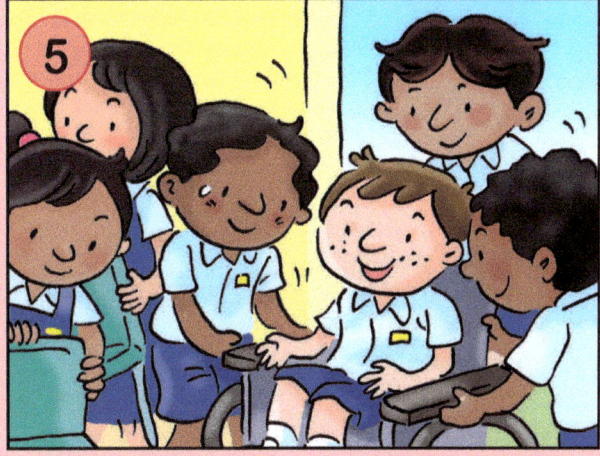

Learning Objective: Pupils will be able to understand different positive and negative emotions experienced.

Sometimes you may feel scared when you are in a new place or with people you do not know. You may feel angry at other times because you wanted to stay where you were.

 What can you do if you are in a new place or with people you do not know? Put a tick (✓) in the boxes.

1
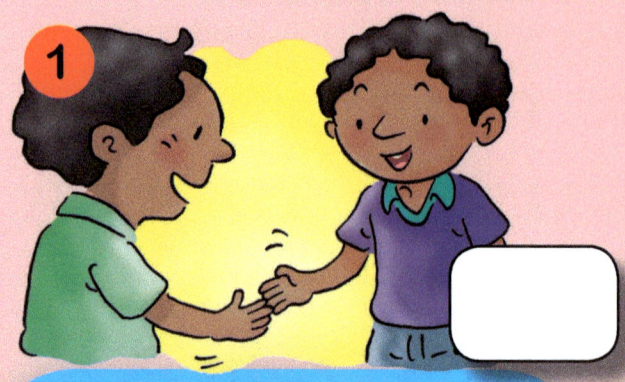
I can try to make friends with someone.

2
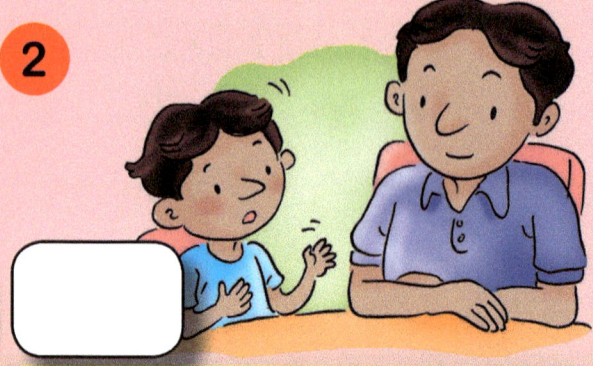
I can talk to a family member about how I feel.

3
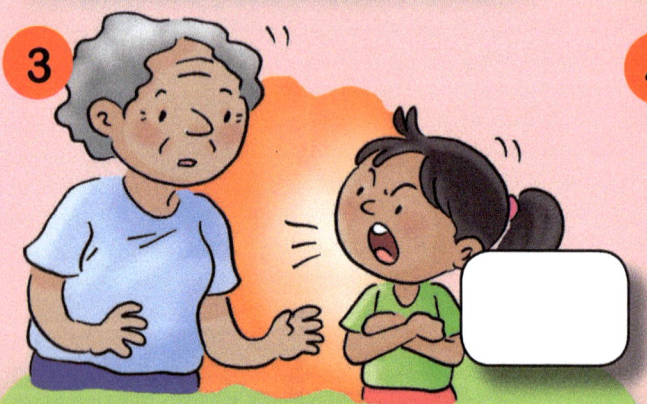
I can shout at others and show how upset I feel.

4
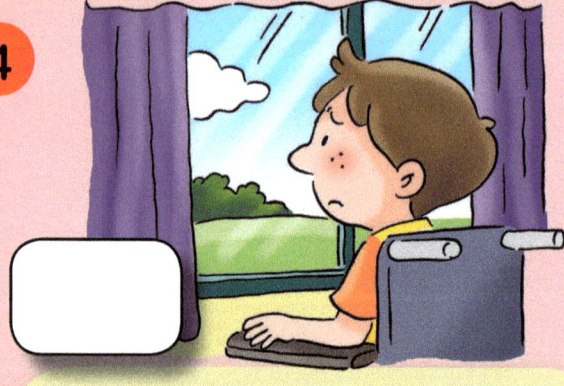
I can hide in my room.

5
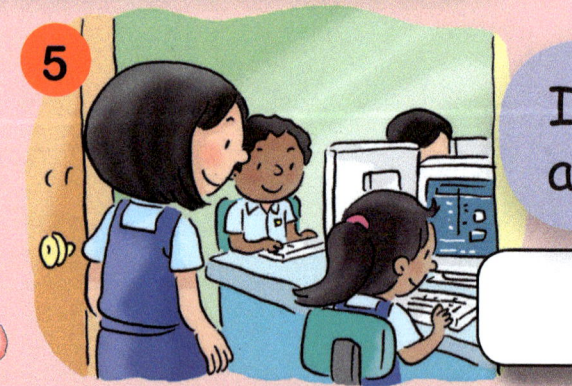
I can take part in an activity I enjoy.

Name: Class: Date: Lessons 4

May I Touch You?

A hug or a pat on the back can make you feel happy and loved. A kick, a punch and tickling can hurt you or make you feel uncomfortable and angry.

Which pictures below show unwanted touches? Put a cross (✗) in the boxes.

1

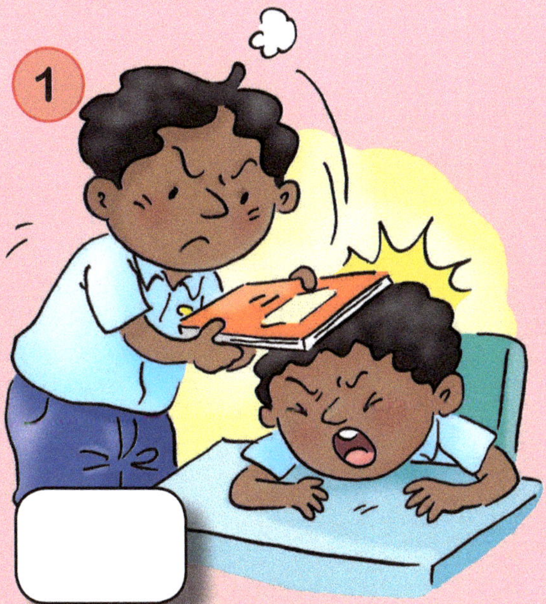

2

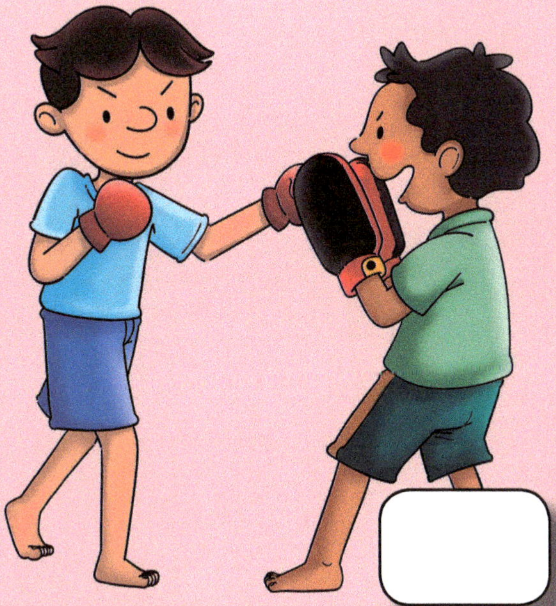

3

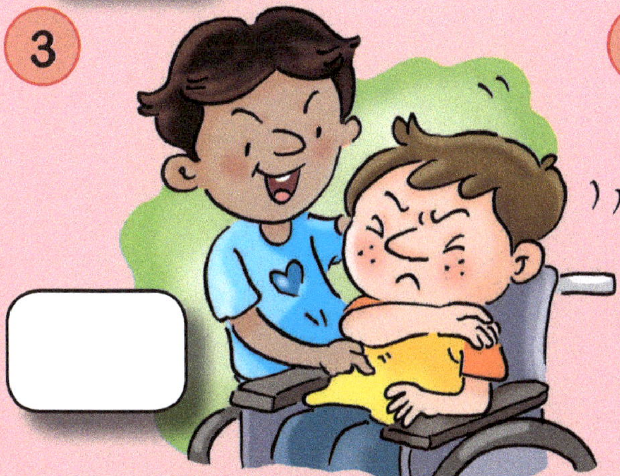

4

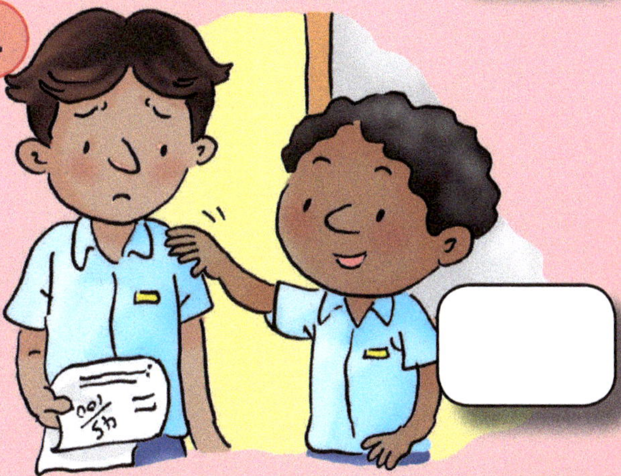

Learning Objective: Pupils will be able to differentiate between good and bad touch.

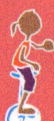 **Draw a red cross (✗) to show where you must not be touched.**

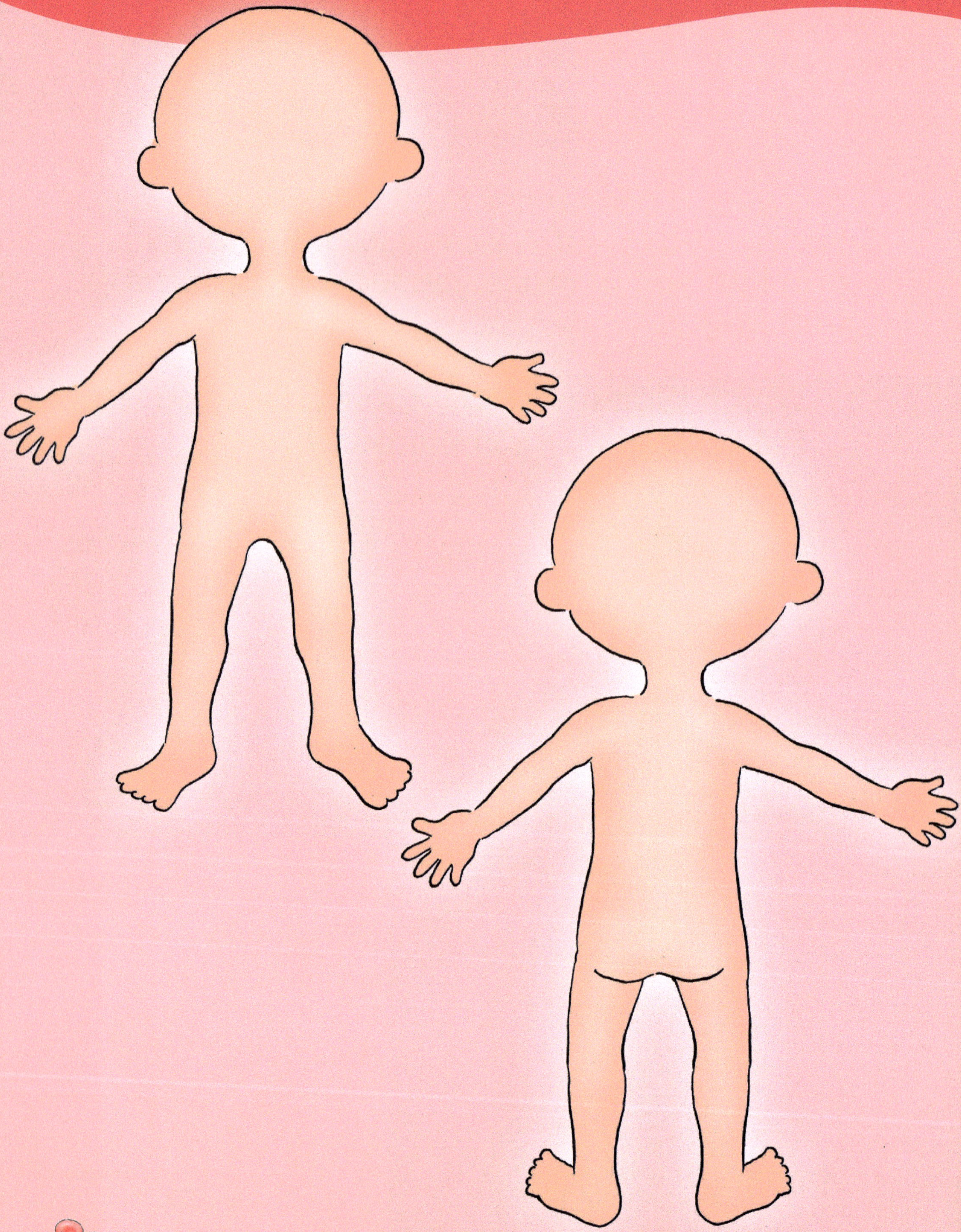

Name: Class: Date: Lesson 5

It Is Not My Fault

Look at the pictures below. Draw lines to match each superfriend to how he or she feels.

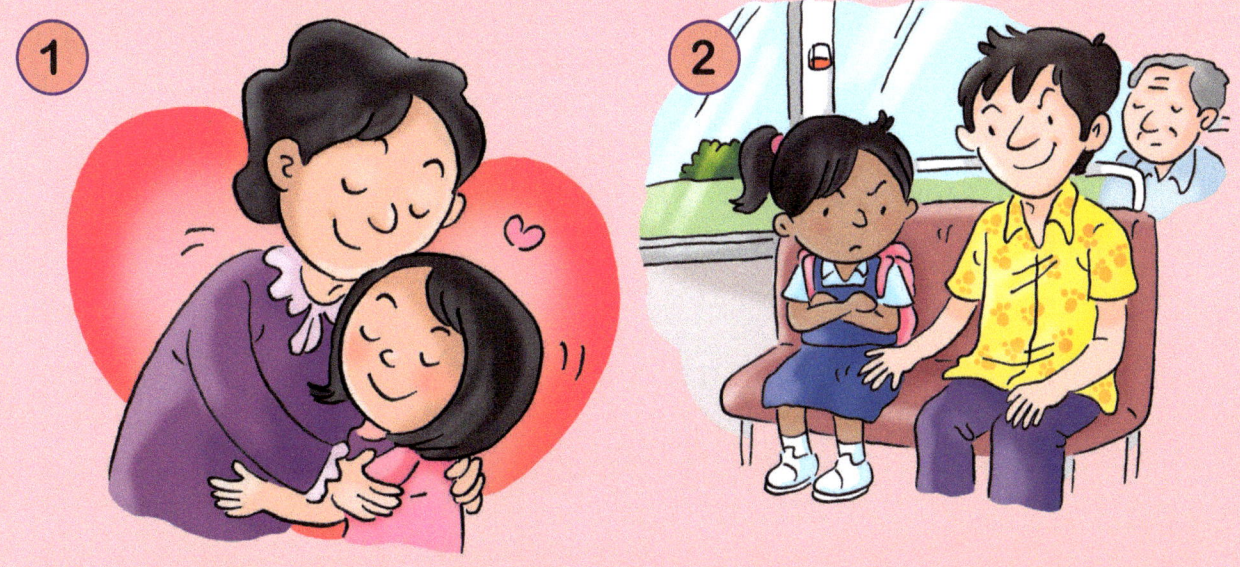

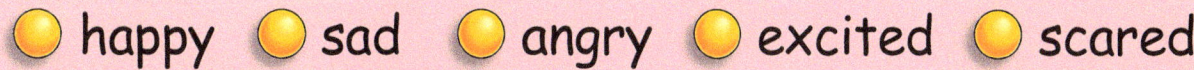
happy   sad   angry   excited   scared

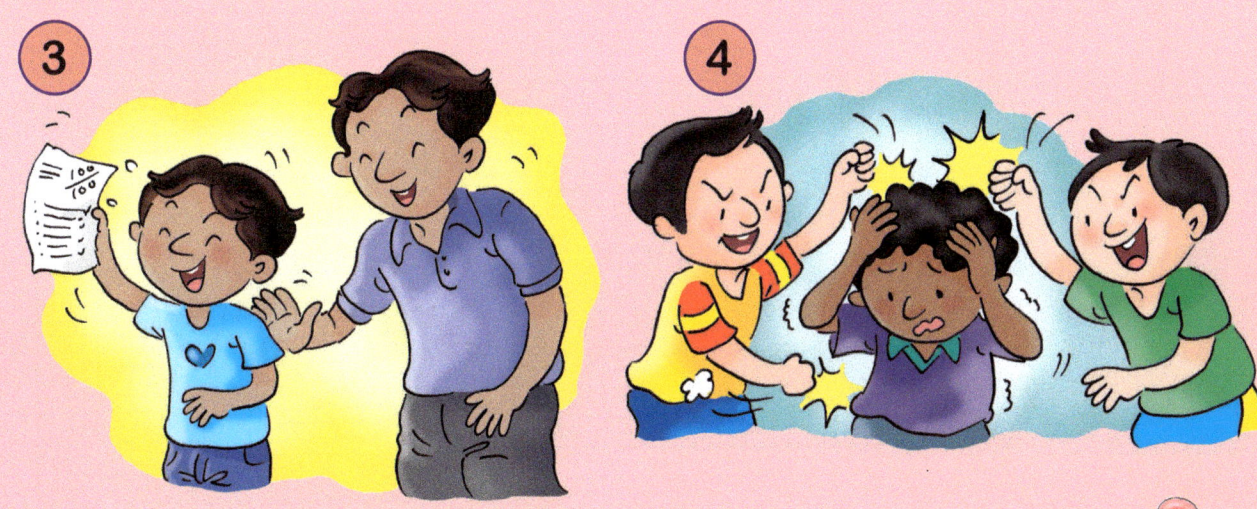

Learning Objective: Pupils will be able to differentiate between good and bad touch.

57

When you receive an unwanted touch, you may think it is your fault. Remember you have not done anything wrong. No one should hurt you or make you feel scared.

Have you ever received an unwanted touch? Put a tick (✓) in 1 and/or 2. Show the places that you have been hurt or touched on the body.

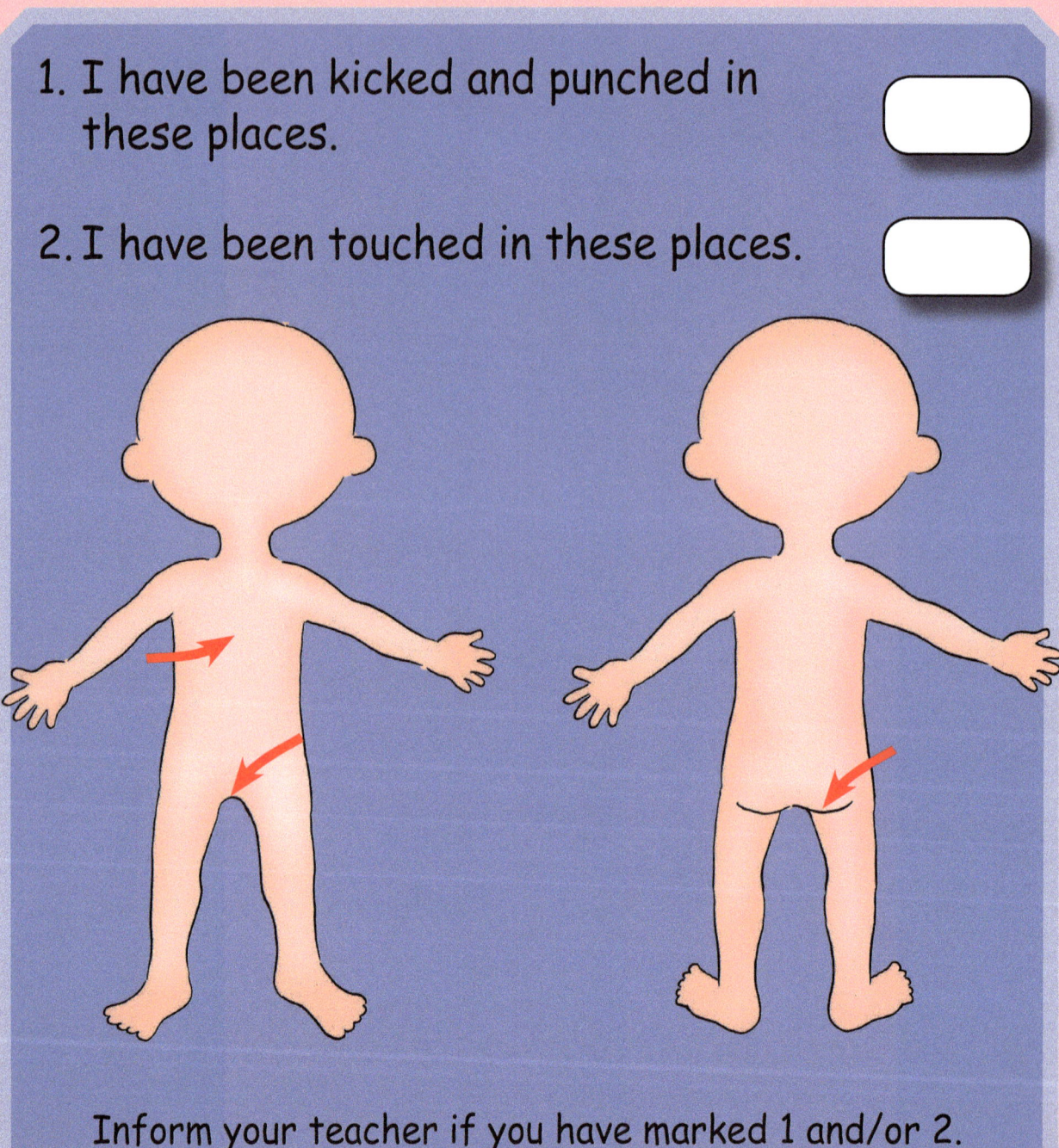

1. I have been kicked and punched in these places.

2. I have been touched in these places.

Inform your teacher if you have marked 1 and/or 2.

Name: Class: Date: Lesson 6

What Can I Do?

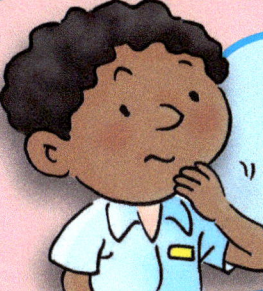

Read what the superfriends are saying.

What will you do if someone tries to hurt you or give you an unwanted touch?

I am not sure. I think I will try to run away!

Hmm... what if I cannot run fast enough?

I am sure she can. She runs faster than I can wheel myself!

I am sure there are better ways of preventing unwanted touches.

What will you do if someone tries to hurt you or give you an unwanted touch?

Learning Objective: Pupils will be able to seek appropriate sources of help or skills needed when threatened by sexual abuse.

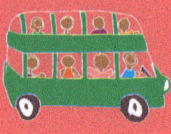 If someone tries to hurt you or give you an unwanted touch, you can say the following to stop him or her.

Stop touching me!

Stop, you are hurting me!

Do not touch me there!

Help! Stop touching and hurting me!

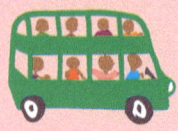 If you hear someone crying for help, this is what you can do. Shout 'Help! Help! Stranger!' until an adult comes.

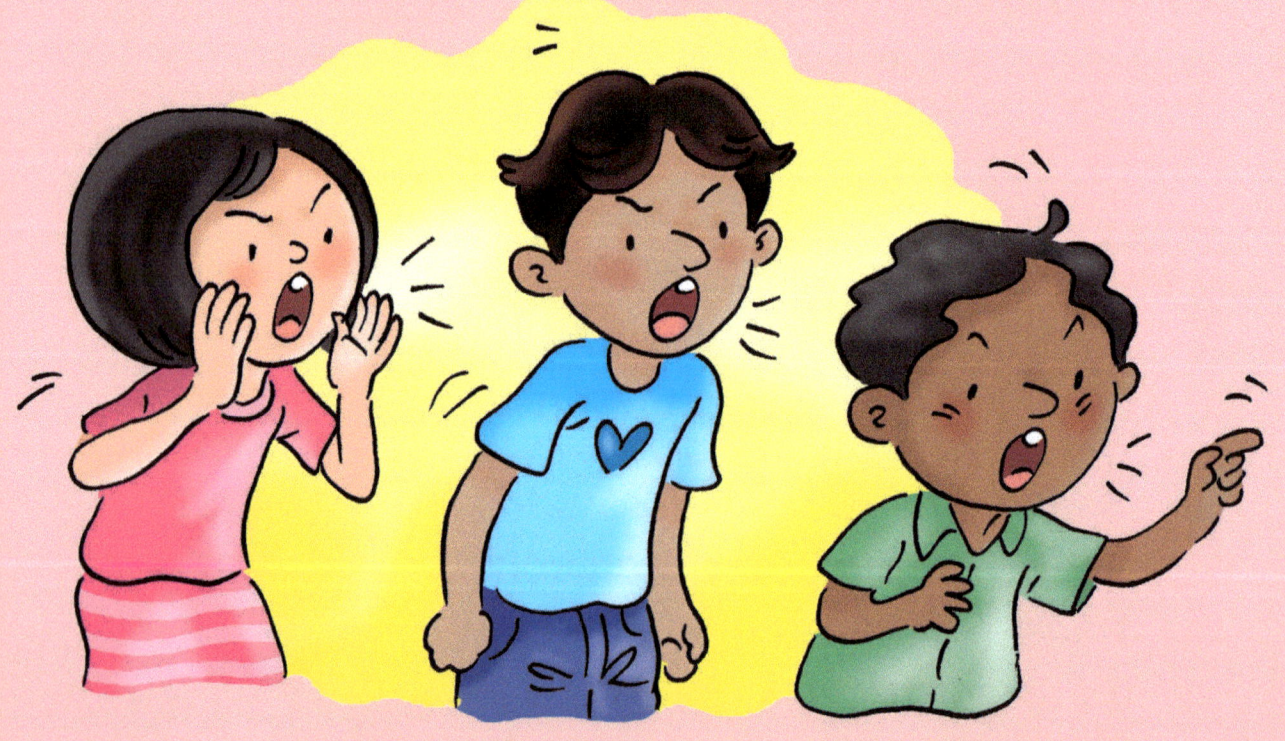

Being Safe At Home

Lesson 7

Name: Class: Date:

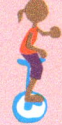 Listen carefully as your teacher reads. Do you think the five superfriends should open the door?
Circle 'Y' for yes and 'N' for no.

1. Should Harold open the door?   Y / N

2. Should Haris open the door?   Y / N

3. Should Lam open the door?   Y / N

4. Should Eileen open the door?   Y / N

5. Should Ajit open the door?   Y / N

Learning Objective: Pupils will be able to seek appropriate sources of help or skills needed when threatened by sexual abuse.

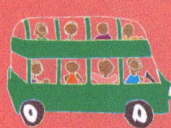

If you are alone at home, keep yourself safe by doing the following.

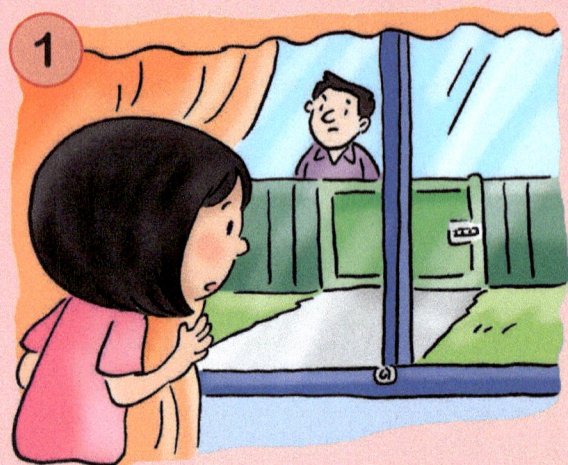

Do not let strangers at the door know you are home alone.

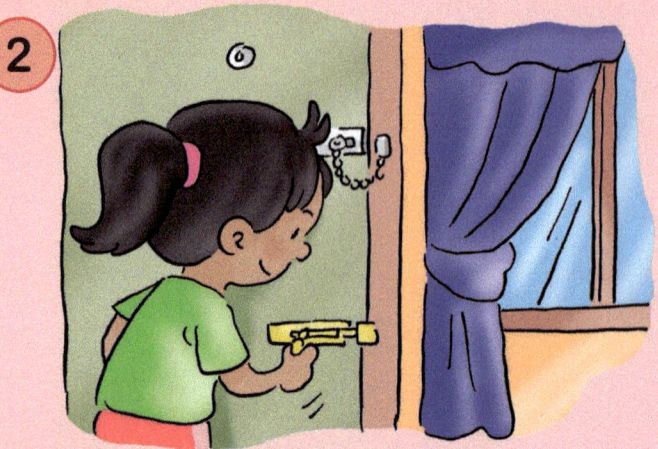

Lock the doors.

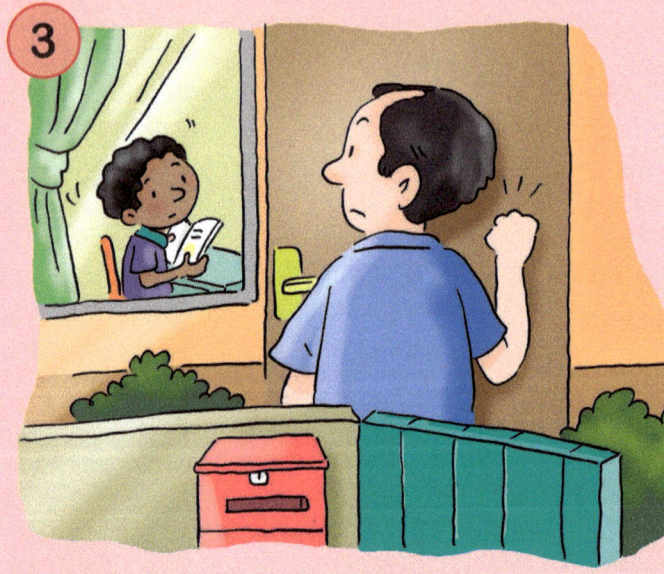

Do not open the door to allow strangers in.

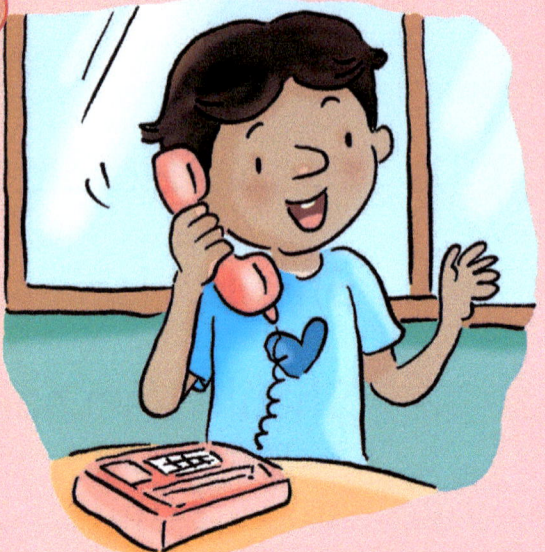

If someone calls and asks for your parents, tell the person your parents are busy and are unable to answer the call.

Remember to always tell an adult you trust about any stranger who tries to enter your home.

Name: Class: Date:

Lesson 8

Being Safe In Public

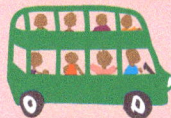 Follow the story in the comic strip below.

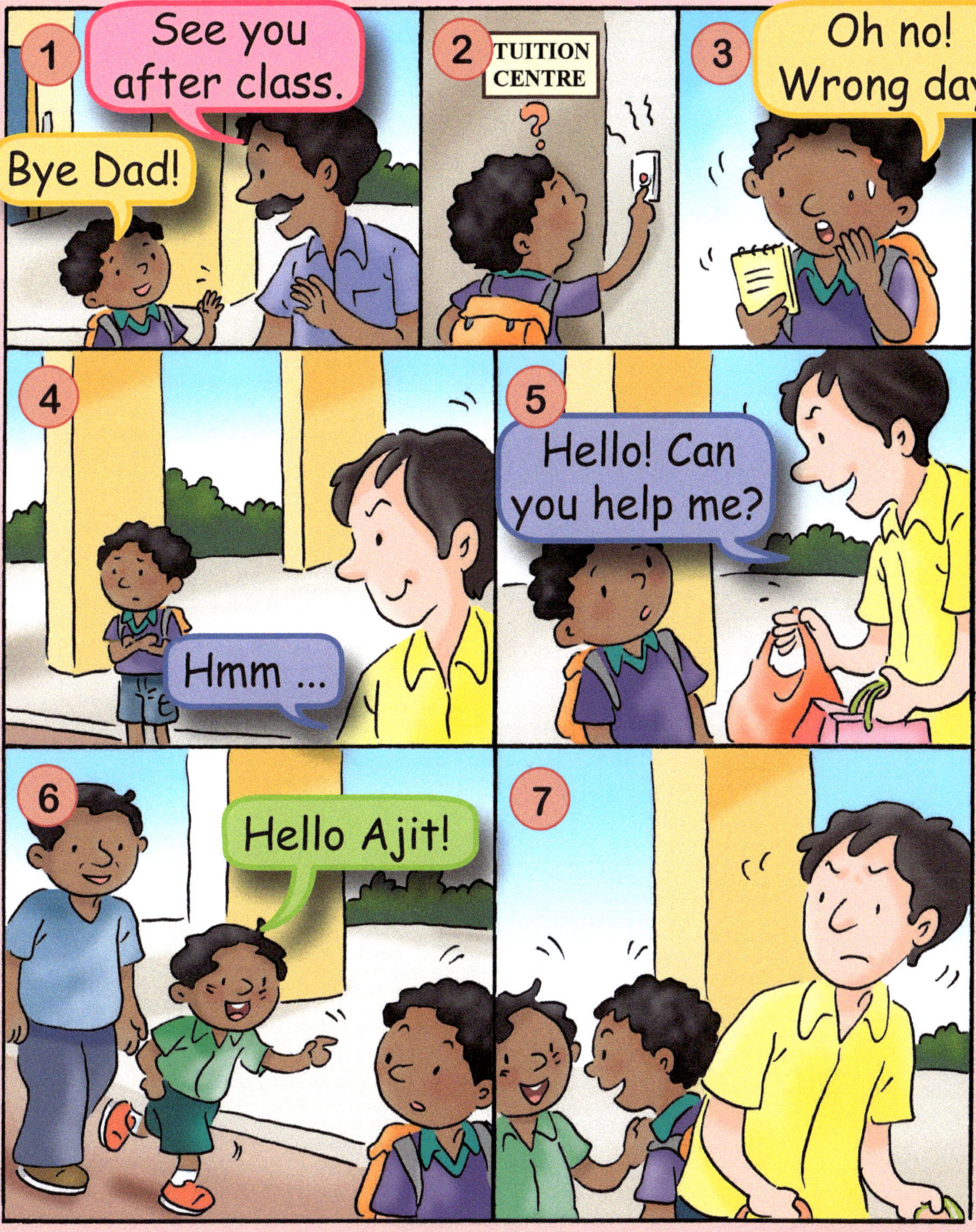

1. Bye Dad! See you after class.

2. TUITION CENTRE

3. Oh no! Wrong day!

4. Hmm ...

5. Hello! Can you help me?

6. Hello Ajit!

7.

Learning Objective: Pupils will be able to seek appropriate sources of help or skills needed when threatened by sexual abuse.

What do you think could have happened to Ajit if he had agreed to help the stranger?

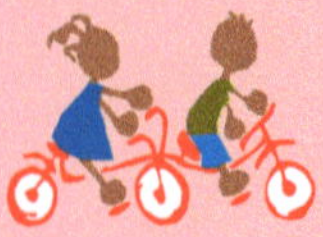

Write your answer below. Use the helping words given.

hurt   harm   rob   wallet   money   missing

_____
_____
_____
_____
_____
_____
_____
_____
_____

NEW WORDS

Lesson: ____ Date: ____

MY LESSON TODAY ...
(Draw or write out the things you remember.)

Lesson: ____ Date: ____

MY LESSON TODAY ...
(Draw or write out the things you remember.)

Lesson: ____ Date: ____

MY LESSON TODAY ...
(Draw or write out the things you remember.)

Lesson: ____ Date: ____

MY LESSON TODAY ...
(Draw or write out the things you remember.)

Lesson: ____ Date: ____

MY LESSON TODAY ...
(Draw or write out the things you remember.)

MY LEARNING LOG

MY LEARNING LOG

NEW WORDS

Lesson: ___ Date: ___

MY LESSON TODAY ...
(Draw or write out the things you remember.)

Lesson: ___ Date: ___

MY LESSON TODAY ...
(Draw or write out the things you remember.)

Lesson: ___ Date: ___

MY LESSON TODAY ...
(Draw or write out the things you remember.)

Lesson: ___ Date: ___

MY LESSON TODAY ...
(Draw or write out the things you remember.)

Lesson: ___ Date: ___

MY LESSON TODAY ...
(Draw or write out the things you remember.)

MY LEARNING LOG

NEW WORDS

Lesson: Date:

MY LESSON TODAY ...
(Draw or write out the things you remember.)

Lesson: Date:

MY LESSON TODAY ...
(Draw or write out the things you remember.)

Lesson: Date:

MY LESSON TODAY ...
(Draw or write out the things you remember.)

Lesson: Date:

MY LESSON TODAY ...
(Draw or write out the things you remember.)

Lesson: Date:

MY LESSON TODAY ...
(Draw or write out the things you remember.)

MY LEARNING LOG

NEW WORDS

Lesson: Date:

MY LESSON TODAY …
(Draw or write out the things you remember.)

Lesson: Date:

MY LESSON TODAY …
(Draw or write out the things you remember.)

Lesson: Date:

MY LESSON TODAY …
(Draw or write out the things you remember.)

Lesson: Date:

MY LESSON TODAY …
(Draw or write out the things you remember.)

Lesson: Date:

MY LESSON TODAY …
(Draw or write out the things you remember.)

NEW WORDS

Lesson: Date:

MY LESSON TODAY ...
(Draw or write out the things you remember.)

Lesson: Date:

MY LESSON TODAY ...
(Draw or write out the things you remember.)

Lesson: Date:

MY LESSON TODAY ...
(Draw or write out the things you remember.)

Lesson: Date:

MY LESSON TODAY ...
(Draw or write out the things you remember.)

Lesson: Date:

MY LESSON TODAY ...
(Draw or write out the things you remember.)

MY LEARNING LOG

MY LEARNING LOG

NEW WORDS

Lesson: _____ Date: _____

MY LESSON TODAY ...
(Draw or write out the things you remember.)

Lesson: _____ Date: _____

MY LESSON TODAY ...
(Draw or write out the things you remember.)

Lesson: _____ Date: _____

MY LESSON TODAY ...
(Draw or write out the things you remember.)

Lesson: _____ Date: _____

MY LESSON TODAY ...
(Draw or write out the things you remember.)

Lesson: _____ Date: _____

MY LESSON TODAY ...
(Draw or write out the things you remember.)